Yoga

AT THE WORK PLACE

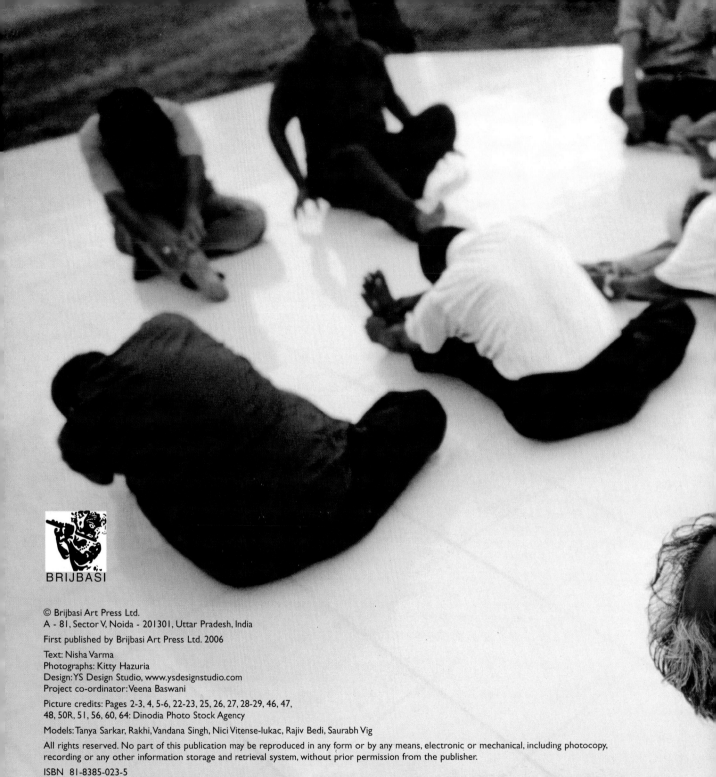

© Brijbasi Art Press Ltd.
A - 81, Sector V, Noida - 201301, Uttar Pradesh, India

First published by Brijbasi Art Press Ltd. 2006

Text: Nisha Varma
Photographs: Kitty Hazuria
Design: YS Design Studio, www.ysdesignstudio.com
Project co-ordinator: Veena Baswani

Picture credits: Pages 2-3, 4, 5-6, 22-23, 25, 26, 27, 28-29, 46, 47,
48, 50R, 51, 56, 60, 64: Dinodia Photo Stock Agency

Models: Tanya Sarkar, Rakhi, Vandana Singh, Nici Vitense-lukac, Rajiv Bedi, Saurabh Vig

ISBN 81-8385-023-5

Processed, printed and bound at Brijbasi Art Press Ltd., A - 81, Sector V, Noida - 201301, Uttar Pradesh, India

Yoga
AT THE WORK PLACE

NISHA VARMA

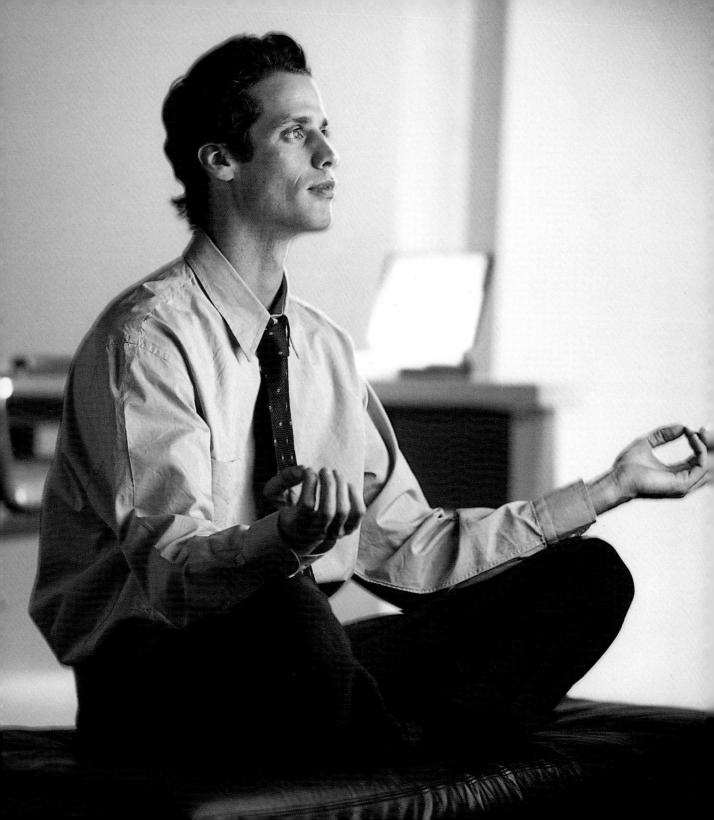

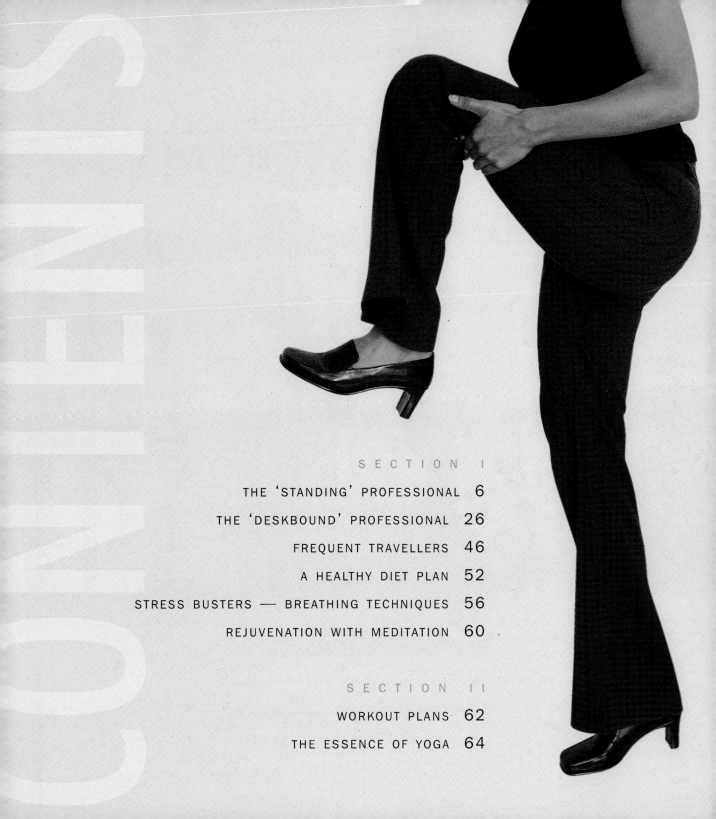

CONTENTS

THE 'STANDING' PROFESSIONAL

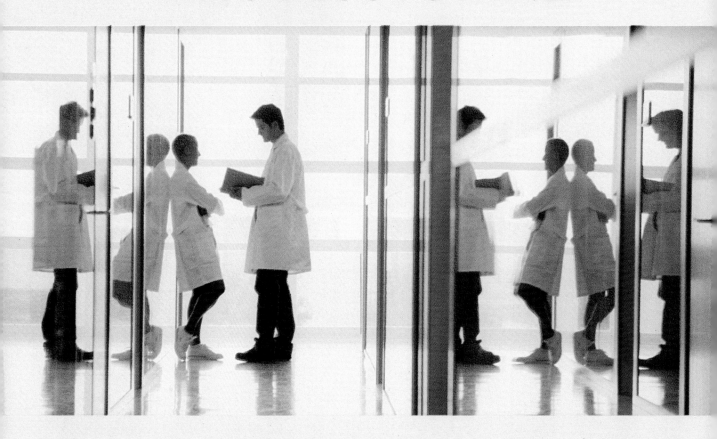

Life moves at a frenetic pace today, what with nuclear families, long hours of work, job pressures, little or no help at home and the necessity to keep up with the overwhelming developing technology around us. How many people are able to take out the time to exercise their bodies and relax their minds? Perhaps only a negligible number. One of the most common complaints you hear is,'By the time I get home, I'm good for nothing else.
All I feel like doing is falling into bed.' Do these words sound familiar?

Gone are the days when people worked mostly in the outdoors,breathed fresh air, and absorbed Vitamin D naturally by soaking in the sunshine. Pollution, adulteration, closed work environments, junk food — all aggravate physical and mental stress. In fact, each profession has its own peculiar hazards:
some require long hours of standing, others involve continuous hours of sedentary work.

To avoid long-term damage to the lower back, avoid wearing high heels
or uncomfortable footwear to work.

Try and sit for short intervals during the day.

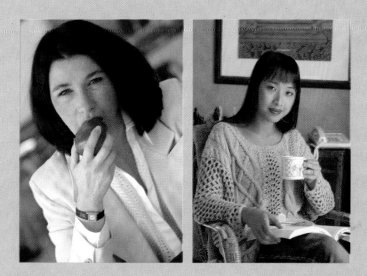

Drink herbal tea two or three times a day. Lemon, jasmine and mint are highly recommended.

Avoid aerated drinks and junk food. Fresh fruits are a good snack food which
not only appease hunger but also keep you feeling light and energetic during the working day.
In fact, five different kinds of fruit are recommended each day.

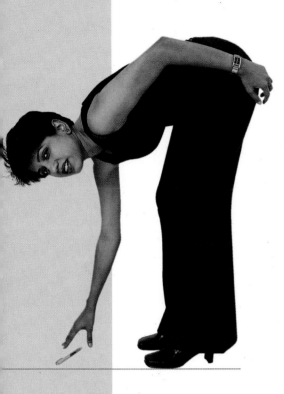

Doctors, lawyers, teachers, shop sales staff, airline cabin crews and people in the hospitality industry, amongst numerous others, have to be on their feet for most of the day. Are you one of them? Are any or several of the following problems faced by you?

- Tending to transfer your weight on to one leg out of exhaustion
- Aching feet and ankles
- Lower back pain
- Nagging pain in the neck and shoulders
- Swollen feet
- Dizzy spells
- Shooting pain from the neck to the arms or legs
- Slouching posture
- Corns, calluses, bunions and ingrown toenails
- Travelling pain in the knee, hipjoints and lower back

'Standing tall' doesn't come so easy any more and you are plagued with aches and pains. Standing over low workstations and constantly bending forward causes stooping shoulders and over-extended muscles of the upper back and neck. Long hours of working in this position can cause compression of the cervical vertebrae and permanent weakness in the muscles of the upper back and neck. Continuous standing on one leg can cause misalignment of the spine and create a permanent defect that can result in a condition similar to Scoliosis, which is usually genetic and in which, the spine could have an extra curve sideways. A person suffering from Scoliosis walks with a peculiar gait as if one leg is shorter than the other. Straining the body more on one side than the other by concentrating the body weight on one leg can lead to permanent damage of the spine. Alignment between the hip and lower back goes awry, resulting in not only a strange-looking body, but extreme lower backache, and fatigue, even when walking short distances.

One of the most common mistakes people make is when they have to do something at the ground level; they tend to bend forward from the hip joint, thus straining the lower back. The sensible way is to kneel on the floor. In fact, the arm muscles should be used for lifting heavy weights instead of straining the lower back. Heavy items such as furniture should never be pushed with the leg or the hip; the arms are meant for such jobs. The arms too often get a beating when excessive weight is hung over one shoulder or carried on one arm. The weight ought to be equally distributed on both shoulders and thus, both sides of the body.

Lack of exercise leads to a weak abdomen, with extra weight around the middle, the belly protrudes and pulls the lower back forward. This creates what is known as a swayback position or Lordosis. An unnatural depression is formed in the lumbar region of the spine, creating a deeper than required lumbar curve and extremely tight muscles and fascia. The result: compression in the lumbar spine and lower backache.

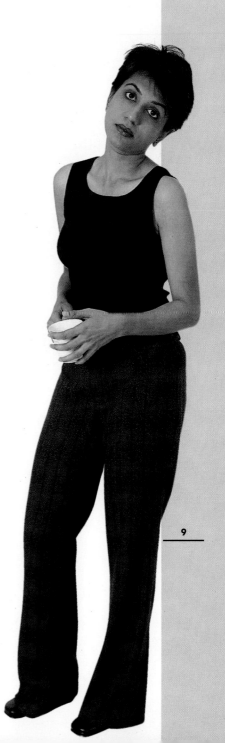

Ill-fitting and high-heeled shoes can damage the multiple tiny bones and delicate muscles and ligaments of the feet and ankles. Chronic ailments can be caused and all perhaps due to standing for long hours in ill-fitting footwear. Shoes should be lightweight, of breathable material, and provide adequate heel, ankle and forefoot support and cushioning. Cheap quality and ill-fitting footwear can lead to deformity in the structure of the foot, leading to permanent damage. If you stand for a long time at work, spare half an hour over weekends to give your feet a good soak in a tub of warm water, followed by a gentle massage with almond oil.

SIMPLE YOGA AT THE WORKPLACE

NECK RELAXATION

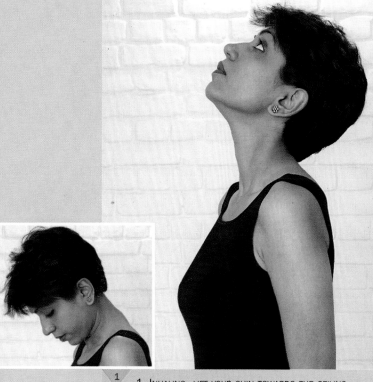

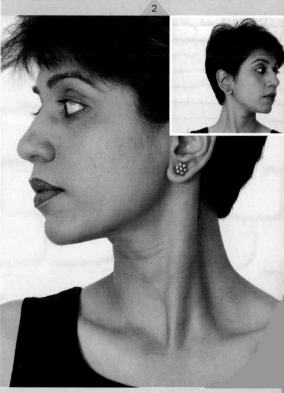

2. TURN THE NECK TOWARDS THE RIGHT SHOULDER AS IF LOOKING OVER THE RIGHT SHOULDER. THIS WILL ALLOW THE MUSCLES IN THE LEFT SIDE OF THE NECK TO STRETCH AND RELAX.
- REPEAT THE SAME ON THE LEFT SIDE.

DO THIS EXERCISE AT LEAST 6 TO 8 TIMES SLOWLY AND WITHOUT JERKS

1. INHALING, LIFT YOUR CHIN TOWARDS THE CEILING, FEELING THE STRETCH IN THE THROAT.
- HOLD IN THAT POSITION FOR 10 SECONDS.
- RELEASE THE STRETCH WHILE EXHALING.

BEND THE NECK BACK EVERY FEW HOURS OR WHENEVER THE NECK FEELS SORE AND TIRED.

THROAT AND VOCAL CHORDS

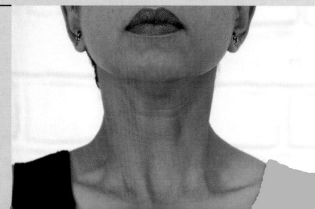

THOSE WHO NEED TO TALK A LOT DURING THE COURSE OF THEIR WORK OFTEN COMPLAIN OF A SORE AND PAINFUL THROAT. THEIR VOICE GETS HOARSE AND NODULES DEVELOP IN THE VOCAL CHORDS.
- INHALE THOUGH THE NOSE.
- HOLD THE BREATH IN AND TIGHTEN THE THROAT AREA. THE VOCAL CHORDS WILL BE PUSHED TIGHT AND FORWARD.
- RELEASE AFTER 6 SECONDS, EXHALING.

REPEAT FOUR TIMES AND DO THIS EXERCISE ONLY TWICE A DAY BUT NOT IMMEDIATELY AFTER A MEAL.

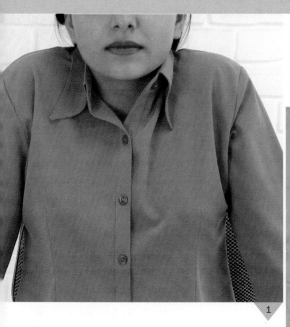

3. INTERLOCK THE HANDS AND LIFT THEM OVERHEAD, GIVING THE MUSCLES OF THE ARMS AND SHOULDERS A GOOD STRETCH.

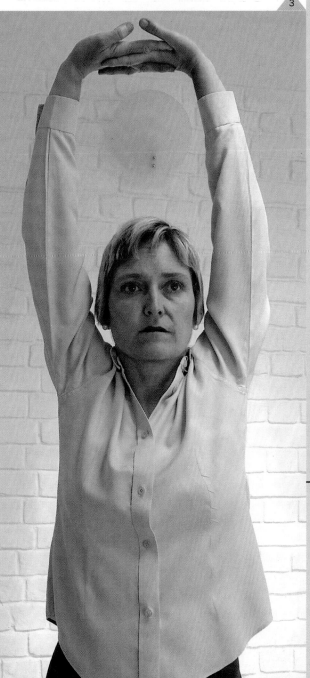

1. LIFT THE SHOULDERS HIGH TOWARDS THE EARS AND LET THEM FALL DOWN GENTLY. REPEAT SEVERAL TIMES DURING THE WORKING DAY.

THIS NOT ONLY RELAXES THE SHOULDER JOINTS BUT THE ARMS AS WELL.

2. ROTATE THE SHOULDERS IN BIG CIRCLES BY FIRST LIFTING THEM TOWARDS THE EARS THEN BACK, DOWN AND FORWARD. REPEAT AT LEAST 8 TIMES WITH THE BACKWARD MOVE AND THEN 8 TIMES STARTING WITH THE FORWARD MOVE.

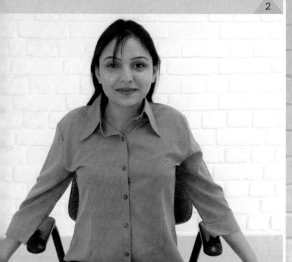

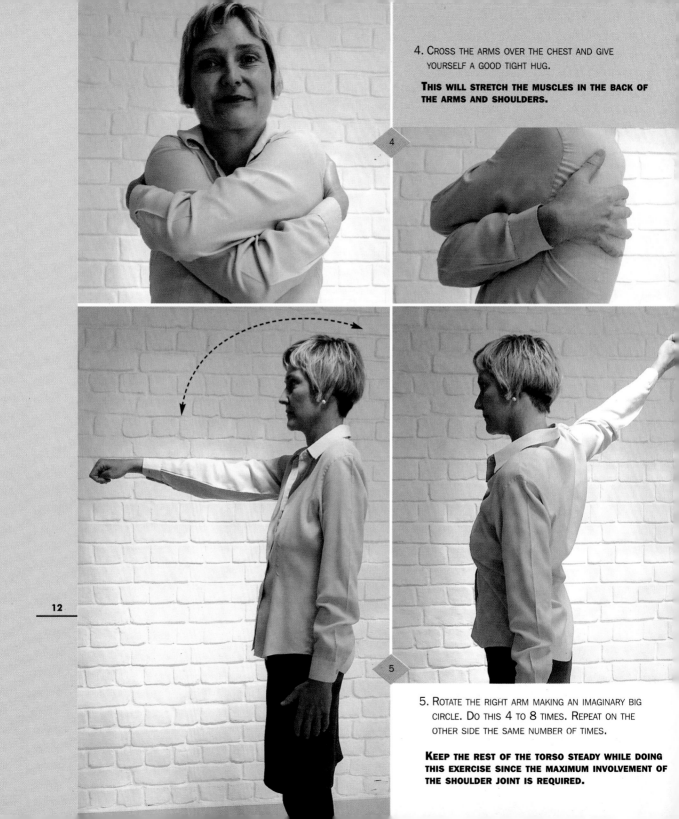

4. CROSS THE ARMS OVER THE CHEST AND GIVE YOURSELF A GOOD TIGHT HUG.

THIS WILL STRETCH THE MUSCLES IN THE BACK OF THE ARMS AND SHOULDERS.

4

5

5. ROTATE THE RIGHT ARM MAKING AN IMAGINARY BIG CIRCLE. DO THIS 4 TO 8 TIMES. REPEAT ON THE OTHER SIDE THE SAME NUMBER OF TIMES.

KEEP THE REST OF THE TORSO STEADY WHILE DOING THIS EXERCISE SINCE THE MAXIMUM INVOLVEMENT OF THE SHOULDER JOINT IS REQUIRED.

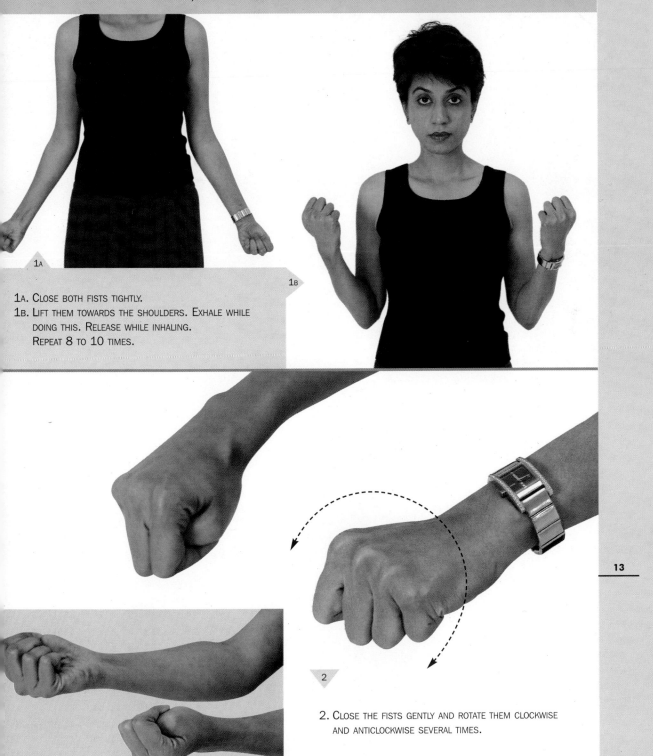

1A. CLOSE BOTH FISTS TIGHTLY.

1B. LIFT THEM TOWARDS THE SHOULDERS. EXHALE WHILE
DOING THIS. RELEASE WHILE INHALING.
REPEAT 8 TO 10 TIMES.

2. CLOSE THE FISTS GENTLY AND ROTATE THEM CLOCKWISE
AND ANTICLOCKWISE SEVERAL TIMES.

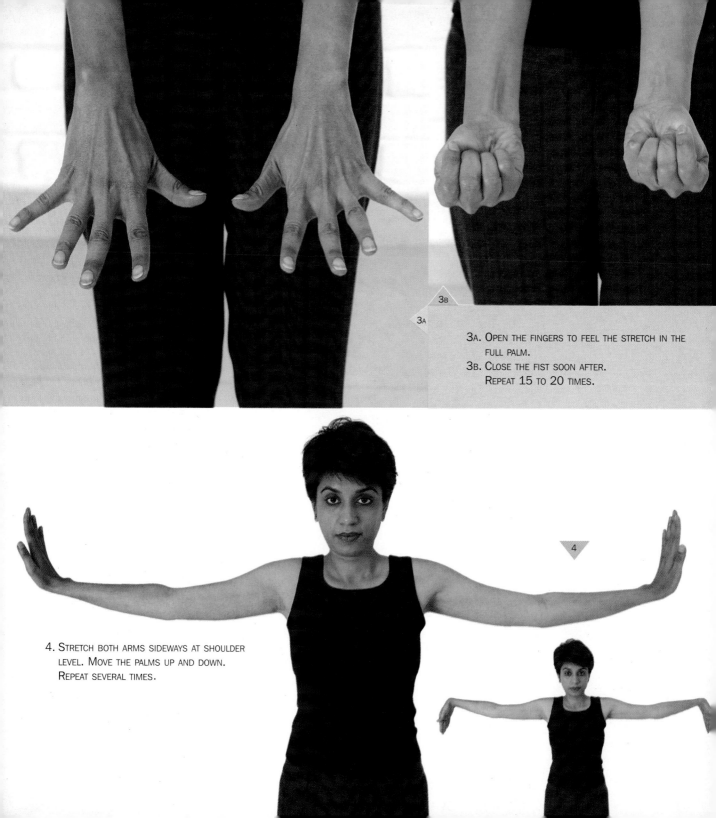

3A. OPEN THE FINGERS TO FEEL THE STRETCH IN THE
FULL PALM.

3B. CLOSE THE FIST SOON AFTER.
REPEAT 15 TO 20 TIMES.

4. STRETCH BOTH ARMS SIDEWAYS AT SHOULDER
LEVEL. MOVE THE PALMS UP AND DOWN.
REPEAT SEVERAL TIMES.

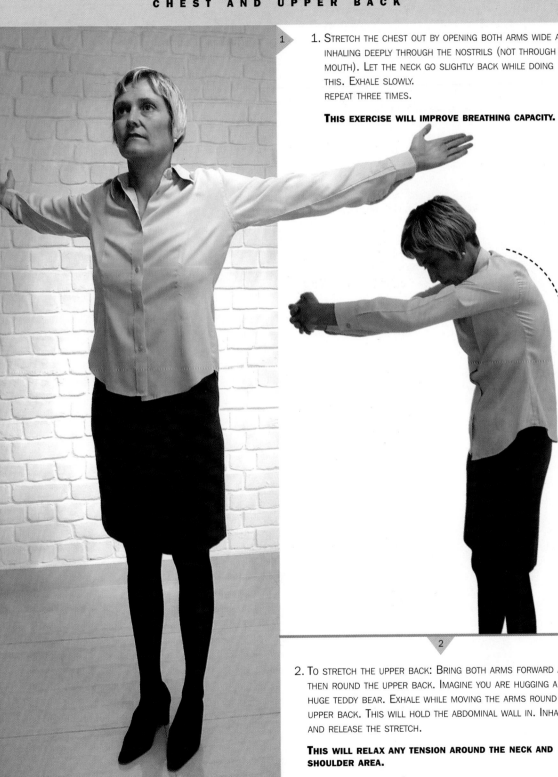

1. STRETCH THE CHEST OUT BY OPENING BOTH ARMS WIDE AND INHALING DEEPLY THROUGH THE NOSTRILS (NOT THROUGH THE MOUTH). LET THE NECK GO SLIGHTLY BACK WHILE DOING THIS. EXHALE SLOWLY.
REPEAT THREE TIMES.

THIS EXERCISE WILL IMPROVE BREATHING CAPACITY.

2. TO STRETCH THE UPPER BACK: BRING BOTH ARMS FORWARD AND THEN ROUND THE UPPER BACK. IMAGINE YOU ARE HUGGING A HUGE TEDDY BEAR. EXHALE WHILE MOVING THE ARMS ROUND THE UPPER BACK. THIS WILL HOLD THE ABDOMINAL WALL IN. INHALE AND RELEASE THE STRETCH.

THIS WILL RELAX ANY TENSION AROUND THE NECK AND SHOULDER AREA.

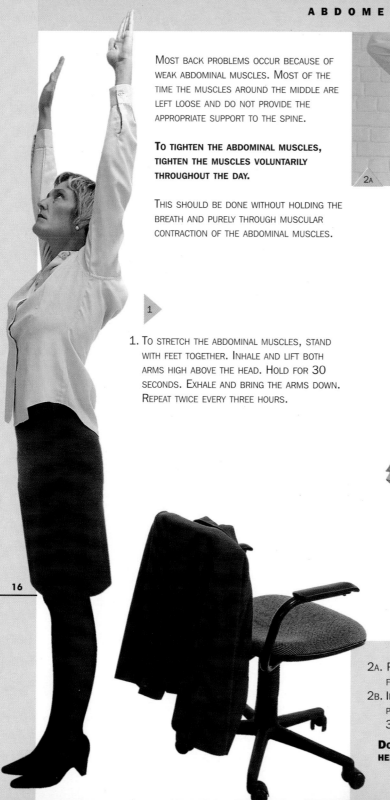

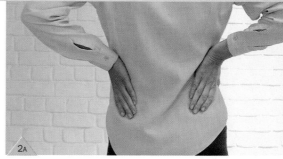

Most back problems occur because of weak abdominal muscles. Most of the time the muscles around the middle are left loose and do not provide the appropriate support to the spine.

TO TIGHTEN THE ABDOMINAL MUSCLES, TIGHTEN THE MUSCLES VOLUNTARILY THROUGHOUT THE DAY.

This should be done without holding the breath and purely through muscular contraction of the abdominal muscles.

1. To stretch the abdominal muscles, stand with feet together. Inhale and lift both arms high above the head. Hold for 30 seconds. Exhale and bring the arms down. Repeat twice every three hours.

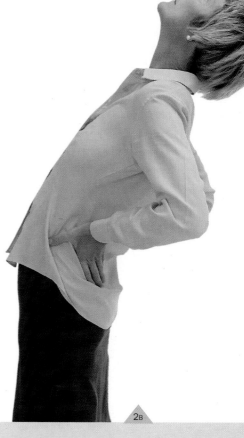

16

2A. Place both hands on the lower back, thumbs forward, remaining fingers at the back.

2B. Inhaling, bend backwards from the waist. Push the pelvis slightly forward while doing this. Hold for 30 seconds. Exhale while returning to position.

DO THIS AS OFTEN AS YOU WISH. EACH TIME THIS WILL HELP TO RELEASE PRESSURE ON THE LOWER BACK.

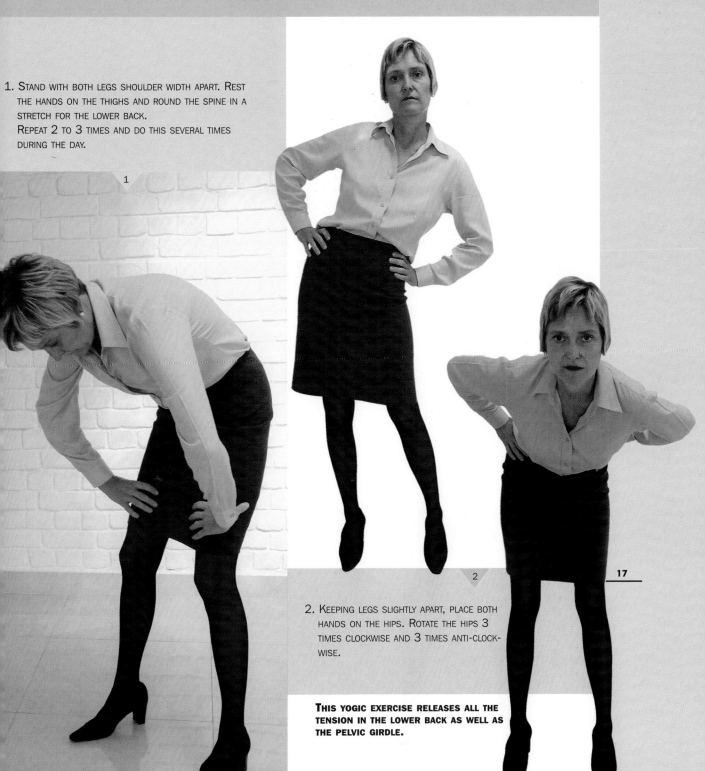

1. STAND WITH BOTH LEGS SHOULDER WIDTH APART. REST THE HANDS ON THE THIGHS AND ROUND THE SPINE IN A STRETCH FOR THE LOWER BACK.
REPEAT 2 TO 3 TIMES AND DO THIS SEVERAL TIMES DURING THE DAY.

1

2

17

2. KEEPING LEGS SLIGHTLY APART, PLACE BOTH HANDS ON THE HIPS. ROTATE THE HIPS 3 TIMES CLOCKWISE AND 3 TIMES ANTI-CLOCK-WISE.

THIS YOGIC EXERCISE RELEASES ALL THE TENSION IN THE LOWER BACK AS WELL AS THE PELVIC GIRDLE.

1A. THIS IS A TWISTING POSTURE AND A SIMPLE WAY TO EXERCISE THE SPINAL VERTEBRAE. STAND WITH LEGS APART. PLACE HANDS ON THE WAIST.

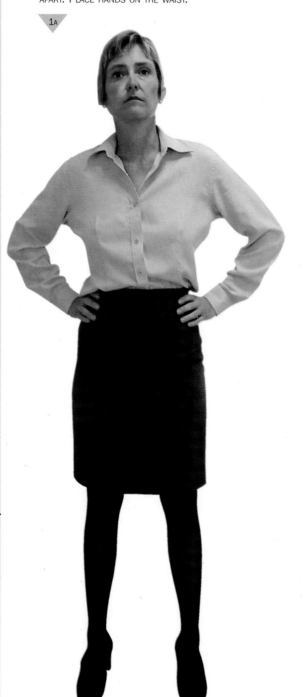

1A

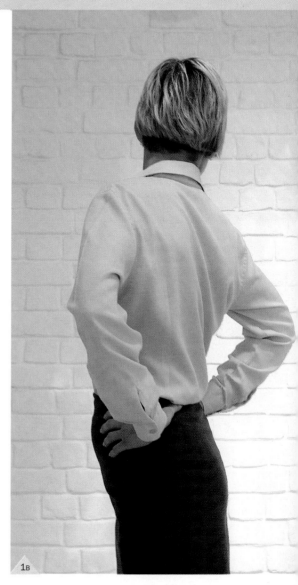

1B

1B. TWIST THE TORSO TOWARDS THE RIGHT, KEEPING YOUR FEET FIRMLY PLANTED ON THE GROUND. INHALE WHILE TURNING BACK.

• EXHALE WHILE TURNING FORWARD.
REPEAT ON THE OTHER SIDE AS WELL. REPEAT AT LEAST THREE TIMES ON EACH SIDE AND DO THE EXERCISE 2 TO 3 TIMES A DAY.

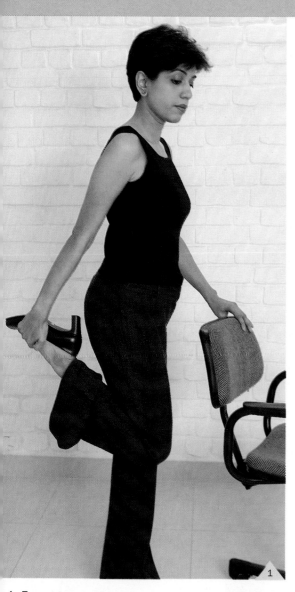

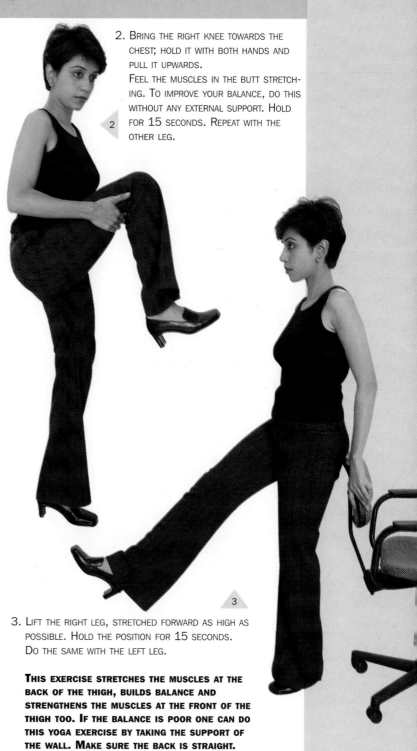

2. BRING THE RIGHT KNEE TOWARDS THE CHEST; HOLD IT WITH BOTH HANDS AND PULL IT UPWARDS.

FEEL THE MUSCLES IN THE BUTT STRETCHING. TO IMPROVE YOUR BALANCE, DO THIS WITHOUT ANY EXTERNAL SUPPORT. HOLD FOR 15 SECONDS. REPEAT WITH THE OTHER LEG.

1. FLEX THE RIGHT LEG BEHIND SO THAT THE ANKLE IS CLOSE TO THE BUTT. HOLD THE RIGHT ANKLE WITH THE RIGHT HAND. FEEL THE STRETCH IN FRONT OF THE THIGH. THE RESTING LEG SHOULD BEAR THE BODY WEIGHT AND THE KNEE OF THE RESTING LEG SHOULD BE SLIGHTLY BENT. HOLD THE STRETCH FOR AT LEAST 30 SECONDS. BUILD UP YOUR BALANCE AND DO THIS EXERCISE WITHOUT THE SUPPORT OF THE CHAIR. REPEAT WITH THE LEFT LEG.

THIS STRETCH WILL RELEASE THE TENSION AND PAIN IN THE STRAINED MUSCLES IN FRONT OF THE THIGH.

3. LIFT THE RIGHT LEG, STRETCHED FORWARD AS HIGH AS POSSIBLE. HOLD THE POSITION FOR 15 SECONDS. DO THE SAME WITH THE LEFT LEG.

THIS EXERCISE STRETCHES THE MUSCLES AT THE BACK OF THE THIGH, BUILDS BALANCE AND STRENGTHENS THE MUSCLES AT THE FRONT OF THE THIGH TOO. IF THE BALANCE IS POOR ONE CAN DO THIS YOGA EXERCISE BY TAKING THE SUPPORT OF THE WALL. MAKE SURE THE BACK IS STRAIGHT.

- STAND STRAIGHT, WITH BOTH FEET TOGETHER, ABOUT A FOOT AWAY FROM THE WALL/TABLE/CHAIR.
  PLACE BOTH HANDS ON THE WALL/TABLE/CHAIR AND TAKE THE LEFT LEG BACK (ABOUT TWO FEET BEHIND).
  BEND THE FORWARD KNEE AND KEEP THE LEFT LEG STRAIGHT BEHIND WITH THE HEEL OF THE FOOT ON THE FLOOR.
  THIS WILL STRETCH THE CALF MUSCLES. HOLD FOR AT LEAST 30 SECONDS.
  REPEAT WITH THE RIGHT LEG BACK.

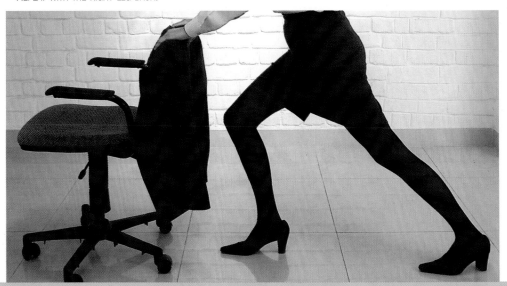

FEET

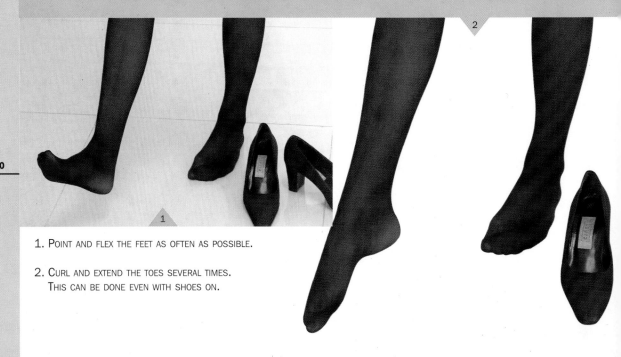

1. POINT AND FLEX THE FEET AS OFTEN AS POSSIBLE.

2. CURL AND EXTEND THE TOES SEVERAL TIMES.
   THIS CAN BE DONE EVEN WITH SHOES ON.

1. RUB BOTH PALMS AGAINST EACH OTHER AND PLACE OVER THE EYES. LEAVE FOR AT LEAST A MINUTE AND THEN REMOVE.

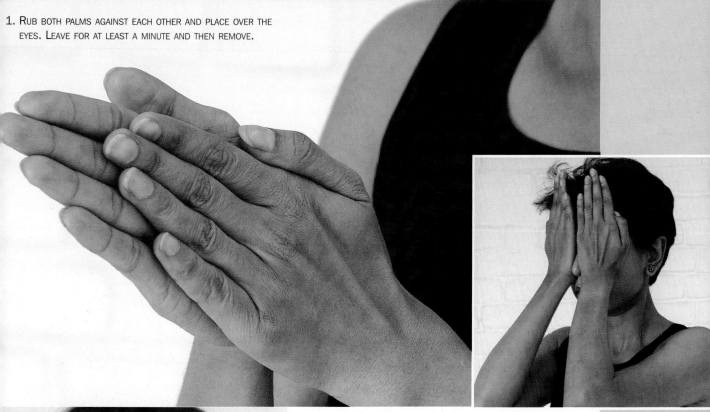

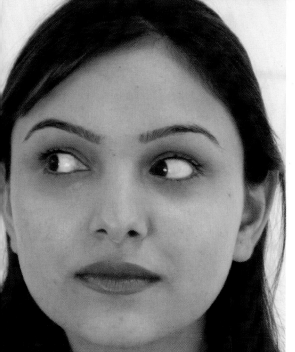

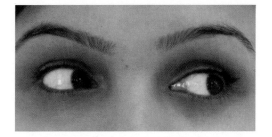

2. MOVE THE PUPILS OF THE EYES FROM RIGHT TO LEFT AT LEAST 8 TIMES.

THIS WILL NOT ONLY HELP THE MUSCLES IN THE EYES TO RELAX BUT WILL RELEASE ANY TENSION AROUND THE FOREHEAD AND TEMPLES.

FIVE-MINUTE MEDITATION

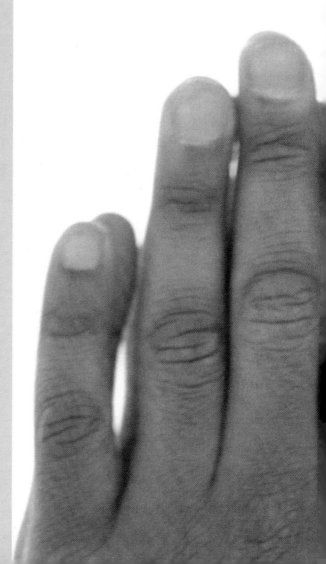

YOGA DOES NOT ONLY PROVIDE PHYSICAL COMFORT. IT IS A WAY OF LIFE THAT INCORPORATES MENTAL, PHYSICAL AND SPIRITUAL WELL-BEING. IT CAN HELP YOU TO LEAD A FOCUSED LIFE AT WORK, AND BE COMPLETELY CENTRED AND RELAXED EVEN WHEN YOU GO HOME AFTER A HARD DAY'S WORK. IT TEACHES YOU TO BE TOLERANT, NON-JUDGEMENTAL AND COMPASSIONATE.

A GREAT WAY TO START YOUR DAY IS WITH A FIVE-MINUTE MEDITATION. THIS CAN BE DONE SOON AFTER WAKING UP.

SIT ON A CHAIR, ON THE BED OR ON A YOGA MAT IN A CROSS-LEGGED POSTURE. MAKE SURE YOUR NECK AND SHOULDERS ARE RELAXED, AND REST YOUR HANDS ON YOUR LEGS/LAP. DO NOT SLOUCH FORWARD. THE LOWER BACK SHOULD REST AGAINST THE BACK OF THE CHAIR OR BE STRAIGHT. CLOSE YOUR EYES AND TAKE A LONG DEEP BREATH IN, EXPANDING THE ABDOMINAL WALL. HOLD THE BREATH FOR A SECOND AND THEN RELEASE IT VERY SLOWLY. FOLLOW THIS PATTERN OF SLOW BREATHING FOR FIVE MINUTES. WITHEVERY EXHALATION, THE BODY SHOULD FEEL HEAVY AND RELAXED.

REPEAT SLOWLY AND STAY STILL FOR AT LEAST FIVE MINUTES BEFORE THE HECTIC PACE OF THE DAY TAKES ITS TOLL ON YOUR MENTAL, PHYSICAL AND SPIRITUAL WELL-BEING.

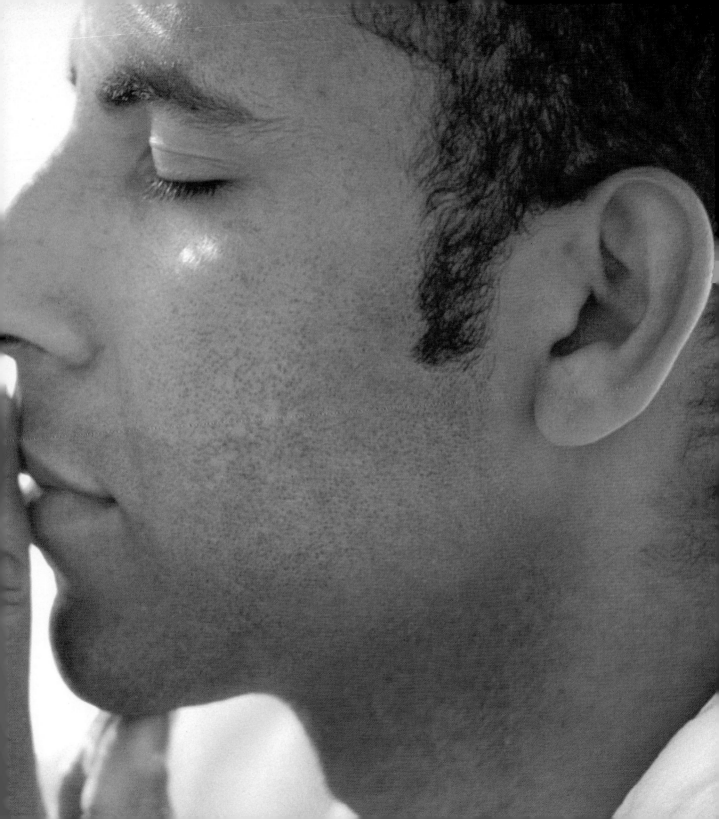

VARICOSE VEINS

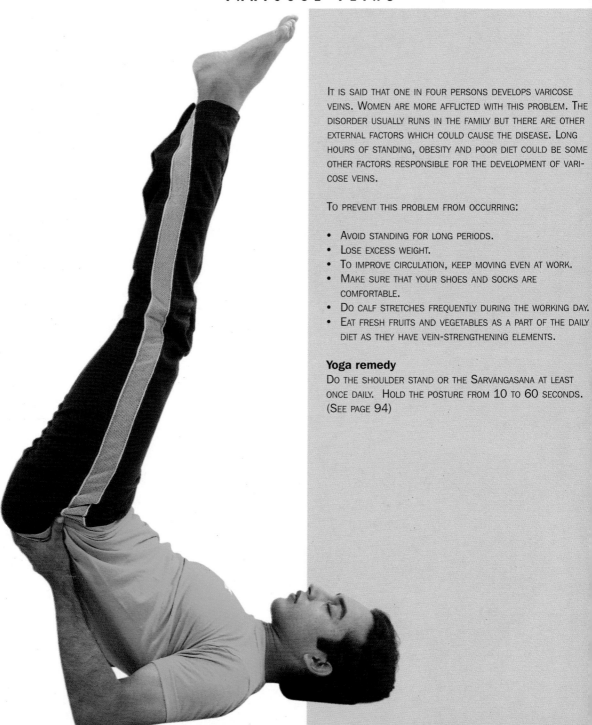

IT IS SAID THAT ONE IN FOUR PERSONS DEVELOPS VARICOSE VEINS. WOMEN ARE MORE AFFLICTED WITH THIS PROBLEM. THE DISORDER USUALLY RUNS IN THE FAMILY BUT THERE ARE OTHER EXTERNAL FACTORS WHICH COULD CAUSE THE DISEASE. LONG HOURS OF STANDING, OBESITY AND POOR DIET COULD BE SOME OTHER FACTORS RESPONSIBLE FOR THE DEVELOPMENT OF VARICOSE VEINS.

TO PREVENT THIS PROBLEM FROM OCCURRING:

- AVOID STANDING FOR LONG PERIODS.
- LOSE EXCESS WEIGHT.
- TO IMPROVE CIRCULATION, KEEP MOVING EVEN AT WORK.
- MAKE SURE THAT YOUR SHOES AND SOCKS ARE COMFORTABLE.
- DO CALF STRETCHES FREQUENTLY DURING THE WORKING DAY.
- EAT FRESH FRUITS AND VEGETABLES AS A PART OF THE DAILY DIET AS THEY HAVE VEIN-STRENGTHENING ELEMENTS.

Yoga remedy

DO THE SHOULDER STAND OR THE SARVANGASANA AT LEAST ONCE DAILY. HOLD THE POSTURE FROM 10 TO 60 SECONDS. (SEE PAGE 94)

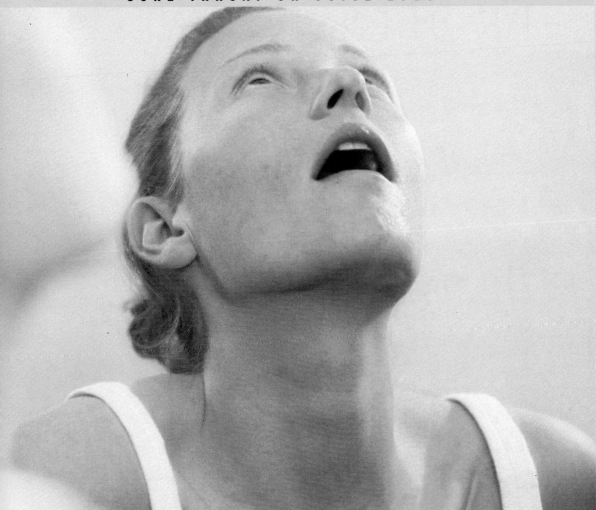

SORE THROAT OR VOICE LOSS IS RELATED TO ANY DISORDER OF THE VOCAL CHORDS WHERE THE NORMAL SPEECH IS DISTURBED AND THE VOICE LOSS COULD BE COMPLETE OR PARTIAL. TEACHERS, SINGERS AND LAWYERS SUFFER FROM AILMENTS OF THE THROAT FREQUENTLY. VOICE LOSS OCCURS WHEN THE VOCAL CHORDS IN THE LARYNX ARE INFLAMED DUE TO AN INFECTION OR DUE TO OVERUSE. NODULES CAN DEVELOP ON THE VOCAL CHORDS IN EXTREME CASES AND MAY REQUIRE SURGERY.

TO PREVENT GREATER DAMAGE TO THE VOICE BOX:
- REST THE VOCAL CHORDS.
- DO NOT SHOUT BUT TALK SOFTLY.
- DRINK FLUIDS BUT NO COFFEE OR ALCOHOL WHICH CAN SERVE AS IRRITANTS RATHER THAN HEALERS.
- AVOID SMOKING OR CHEWING TOBACCO.
- GARGLE FREQUENTLY WITH MILDLY SALTED LUKEWARM WATER.

THE 'DESKBOUND' PROFESSIONAL

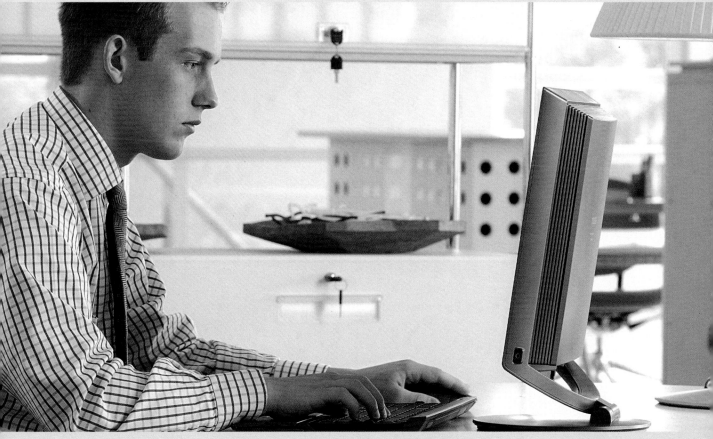

For most people with deskbound jobs, a normal working day comprises at least ten to fourteen hours, six days a week. There are some who do not even look away from their files or computer screens for hours together and the strain results in:

• Headaches • Cervical problems • Carpal tunnel Syndrome • Fast failing eyesight • Nausea • Indigestion/ lack of appetite/hyperacidity • Weight gain • Weak lower body muscles • Weak pelvic floor muscles • Pot belly • Decreased lumbar curve resulting in lower backache • Stiffness in the calves • Burning in the soles of the feet • Poor circulation of blood

Pain in the joints • Reduced range of movement or stiff and painful joints

Long working hours at the desk leave you feeling dull and listless most of the time. Day after day the hectic work schedules, deadlines and other work-related hassles leave little or no energy to cope with anything else. Relationships and domestic responsibilities suffer as does physical well-being. An hour's workout everyday is next to impossible and Sundays are normally spent trying to catch up with sleep and housework. With less time and more work the stress levels are high as well, and stress-related diseases are the bane of the urban professional. However, the solution is simple and fitness can be achieved in small measures during the working day to get a cumulative fitness benefit. Holidays and weekends can be devoted to a longer yoga regime and to games like tennis, squash, golf or other forms of exercise like swimming, jogging or walking.

STRETCH AND SHRUG

1. START THE DAY WITH A STRETCH. STAND WITH BOTH FEET TOGETHER AND BREATHE DEEPLY, TAKING BOTH ARMS OVERHEAD. LOOK UP AND S_T_R_E_T_C_H. DO THIS TWO OR THREE TIMES.

2. NEXT, SHRUG BOTH SHOULDERS SEVERAL TIMES AND THEN ROTATE THEM SEVERAL TIMES.

3. CROSS BOTH ARMS OVER THE CHEST AND GIVE YOURSELF A GOOD HUG.

4. TAKE A FEW LONG DEEP BREATHS IN, EXPANDING THE ABDOMEN WHILE INHALING AND RELAX THE WHOLE BODY WHILE EXHALING.

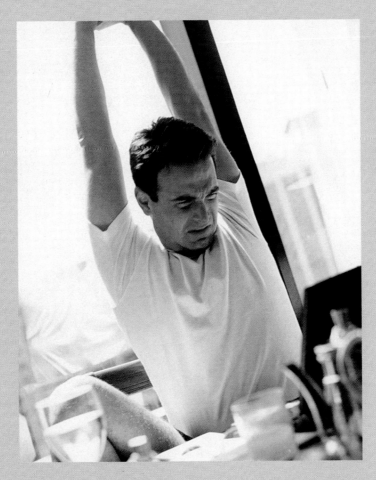

THESE SIMPLE EXERCISES WILL HELP YOU LIMBER UP, START THE DAY WITH VIGOUR AND RELEASE STIFF JOINTS AND MUSCLES.

IMPROVE CIRCULATION

Poor circulation is a result of lack of physical activity and can result in:

- Muscle fatigue
- Lack of energy
- Poor skin tone
- Listless hair
- Inadequate oxygen in the body

For people with a sedentary job, it is very important to move around as much as possible during the day to improve the circulatory system. A conscious effort needs to be made to incorporate physical activity in your working day. To improve circulatory fitness, try adopting the following lifestyle changes:

1. Park the car at least half a kilometre away from the office. Train and bus travellers can get off a couple of stations before the destined stop and walk the rest of the way to office. If all else fails, walk around the office block during the lunch hour (specially in winter).
2. Climb the stairs instead of taking the elevator.
3. Eat breakfast every day to keep the energy levels high in the morning. Make sure it is rich in complex carbohydrates.
4. Avoid excessive intake of coffee. Avoid cigarettes, colas and aerated drinks completely. Drink lots of water and in summer, a glass of juice at around eleven a.m. Buttermilk, tender coconut water or lime juice with a pinch of salt and sugar are refreshing as well as energising drinks. Herbal teas and iced teas (with less sugar) are a good idea as well.
5. Eat a balanced lunch and avoid fried food.
6. Avoid junk food as it will only make you lethargic.

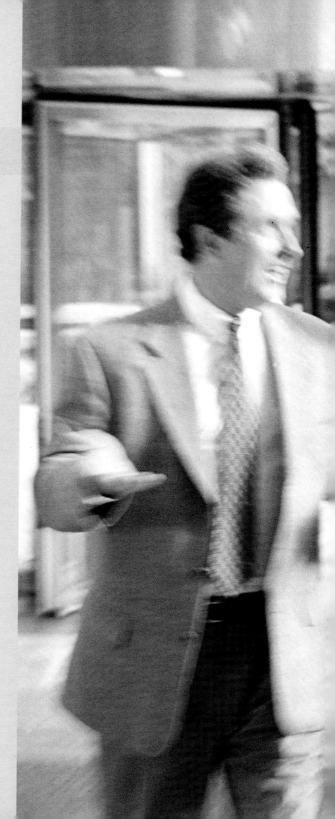

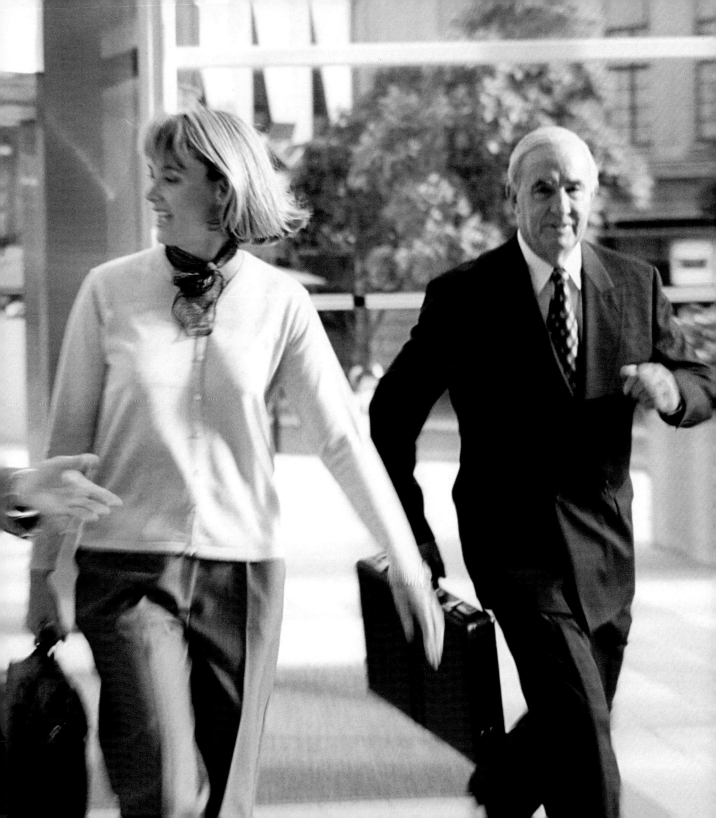

SIMPLE YOGA EXERCISES

STRETCH OUT ON THE TABLE

1. SIT IN THE CHAIR, STRETCH BOTH ARMS ON THE TABLE AND STRETCH THE UPPER BODY BY BENDING FORWARD.

THIS WILL STRETCH THE MUSCLES OF THE BACK, SHOULDERS AND THE ARMS.

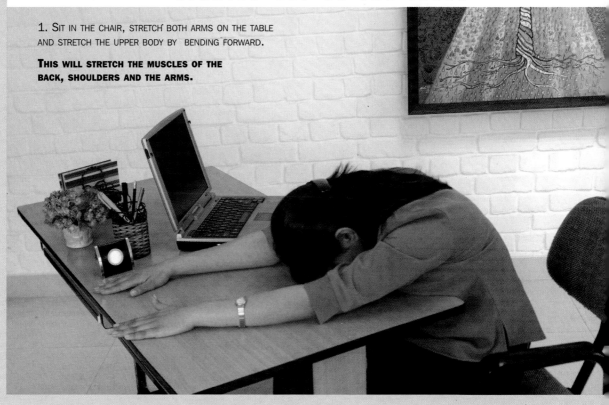

ABDOMEN AND PELVIC MUSCLES

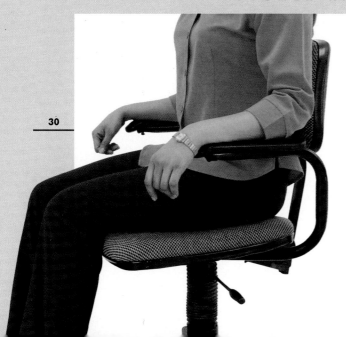

A WEAK ABDOMINAL WALL AND WEAK PELVIC MUSCLES RESULT IN NOT ONLY A PROTRUDING BELLY BUT COULD CAUSE A PERMANENT WEAKNESS OF THE PELVIC MUSCLES WHICH HOLD AND SUPPORT THE ORGANS IN THE PELVIC AREA.

1. **SEATED ABDOMINAL COMPRESSION:** WHILE SITTING AT THE WORKSTATION TRY AND HOLD IN THE LOWER ABDOMINAL AREA AS TIGHTLY AS POSSIBLE FOR AS LONG AS YOU CAN. DO NOT HOLD THE BREATH WHILE DOING THIS. IT SHOULD BE A MUSCULAR CONTRACTION AND WILL HELP TIGHTEN THE ABDOMINAL WALL.

WHILE SITTING TIGHTEN NOT ONLY THE ABDOMINAL MUSCLES BUT ALSO PRESS THE INNER THIGHS TOGETHER, PULLING THE NAVAL TOWARDS THE SPINE TO FEEL A COMPRESSION IN THE LOWER ABDOMINAL AREA.

THESE SIMPLE EXERCISES ARE VARIATIONS OF AN EXERCISE IN YOGA AND STRENGTHEN THE MUSCLES OF THE URINARY AND REPRODUCTIVE ORGANS OF THE BODY. THEY TONE THE ABDOMINAL MUSCLES AND STRENGTHEN THE PELVIC MUSCLES.

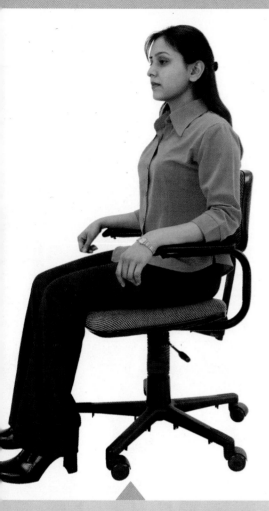

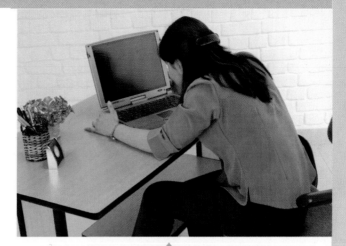

WHILE SITTING, AVOID LEANING FAR FORWARD ON THE DESK BY PLACING BOTH ELBOWS ON THE TABLE AND BUNCHING THE SHOULDERS TOWARDS THE EARS.

THIS CAUSES STRESS ON THE MUSCLES OF THE CERVICAL REGION.

IF WORKING AT A COMPUTER MAKE SURE THE SCREEN IS AT EYE LEVEL.

THIS WILL PREVENT COMPRESSION OF THE CERVICAL VERTEBRAE.

ALWAYS SIT UPRIGHT REGARDLESS OF THE NATURE OF THE WORK. THE NECK AND SHOULDER MUSCLES SHOULD BE RELAXED, WITH THE SHOULDER BLADES PULLED BACK AND DOWN AND CHEST OUT.

IN THIS POSTURE THERE WILL BE NO STRESS ON THE SPINE. SLOUCHING COMES EASY BUT IT GRADUALLY WEAKENS THE SPINE FROM THE CERVICAL TO THE LUMBAR REGION AS THE MUSCLES LOSE STRENGTH.

IF THERE IS TOO MUCH GAP BETWEEN THE LOWER BACK AND THE CHAIR THEN PLACE A CUSHION TO SUPPORT THE SPINE AND MAINTAIN THE NATURAL CURVE IN THE LOWER BACK TO KEEP IT FREE OF STRESS. IDEALLY THE THIGHS SHOULD BE PARALLEL TO THE FLOOR AND THE FEET SHOULD REST COMFORTABLY ON THE FLOOR WITHOUT CAUSING UNDUE STRESS ON THE LOWER OR THE UPPER BACK.

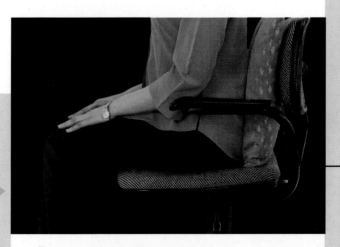

31

FROM A SEATED POSTURE YOU CAN DO VERY LITTLE TO EXERCISE THE BACK OR MOBILISE THE SPINE. TO PREVENT LONG-TERM DAMAGE TO THE SPINE AND PERMANENT WEAKNESS OF THE MUSCLES SURROUNDING AND SUPPORTING THE SPINE, PERFORM THE FOLLOWING EXERCISES AT LEAST ONCE DURING THE COURSE OF A WORKING DAY. AVOID DOING THESE EXERCISES SOON AFTER A MEAL.

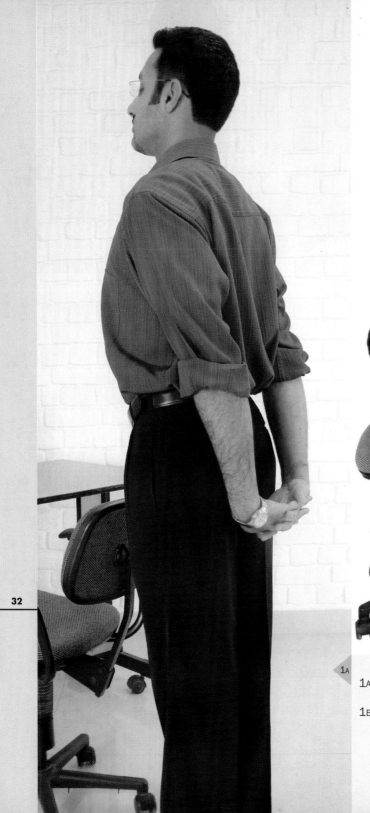

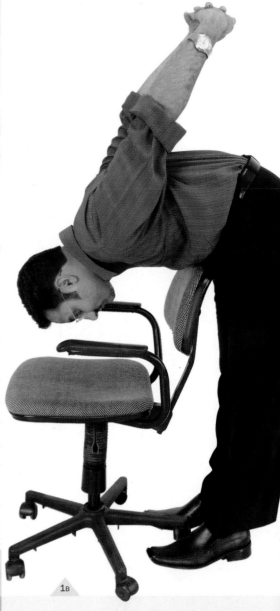

1A.

1B.

1A. STAND BEHIND THE CHAIR AND LOCK BOTH HANDS BEHIND
   THE BACK.
1B. EXHALE AND BEND FORWARD SO THE STOMACH RESTS AGAINS
   THE BACK OF THE CHAIR AND THE ARMS ARE LIFTED HIGH
   BEHIND THE BODY.

**THIS EXERCISE WILL STRETCH THE SPINE ITSELF AS WELL
AS THE MUSCLES OF THE BACK. REPEAT TWICE.**

2. Maintaining the same position as above, bend forward and let the upper body hang loose over the chair. Feel the stretch in the muscles of the upper and the lower back while doing this.

This stretches the muscles of the upper back and relaxes the back. Hold for 30 seconds at least.

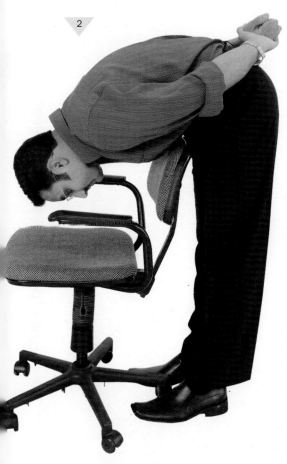

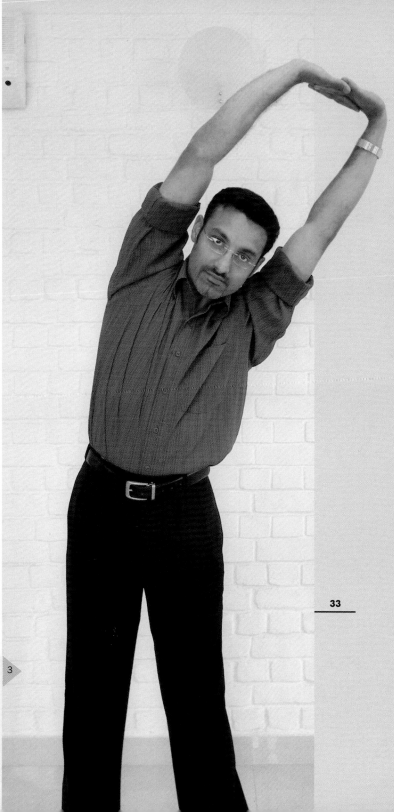

3. From the same starting position, inhale deeply and take both arms overhead and interlock the fingers. Stretch the arms fully towards the ceiling. Exhale and bend laterally towards the left. Make sure not to bend forward. Repeat on the right side and hold each posture for ten to fifteen seconds.

This stretches the sides of the trunk.

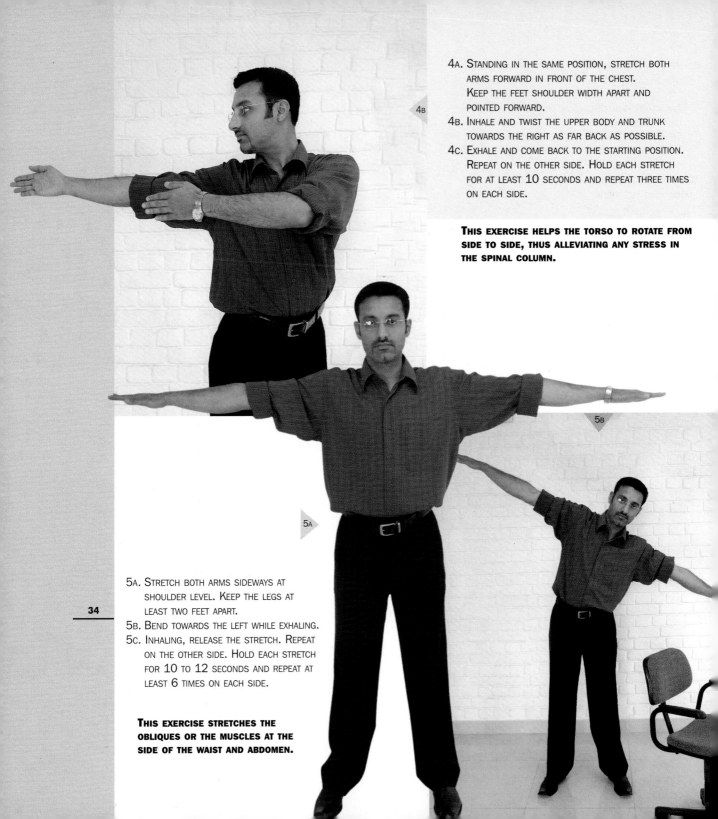

4A. STANDING IN THE SAME POSITION, STRETCH BOTH
ARMS FORWARD IN FRONT OF THE CHEST.
KEEP THE FEET SHOULDER WIDTH APART AND
POINTED FORWARD.

4B. INHALE AND TWIST THE UPPER BODY AND TRUNK
TOWARDS THE RIGHT AS FAR BACK AS POSSIBLE.

4C. EXHALE AND COME BACK TO THE STARTING POSITION.
REPEAT ON THE OTHER SIDE. HOLD EACH STRETCH
FOR AT LEAST 10 SECONDS AND REPEAT THREE TIMES
ON EACH SIDE.

**THIS EXERCISE HELPS THE TORSO TO ROTATE FROM
SIDE TO SIDE, THUS ALLEVIATING ANY STRESS IN
THE SPINAL COLUMN.**

4B

5B

5A

5A. STRETCH BOTH ARMS SIDEWAYS AT
SHOULDER LEVEL. KEEP THE LEGS AT
LEAST TWO FEET APART.

5B. BEND TOWARDS THE LEFT WHILE EXHALING.

5C. INHALING, RELEASE THE STRETCH. REPEAT
ON THE OTHER SIDE. HOLD EACH STRETCH
FOR 10 TO 12 SECONDS AND REPEAT AT
LEAST 6 TIMES ON EACH SIDE.

**THIS EXERCISE STRETCHES THE
OBLIQUES OR THE MUSCLES AT THE
SIDE OF THE WAIST AND ABDOMEN.**

Working for long hours at a computer terminal can take its toll on the health of the eyes. It is essential to ease the stress on the eyes

1A. Look away from the monitor towards some distant object and shift the focus of the eyes frequently.

1B. Then rub both palms together.

1C. close the eyes and place the palms on the eyes. Hold for at least a minute.

THIS WILL RELEASE THE STRESS ON THE DELICATE MUSCLES OF THE EYES.

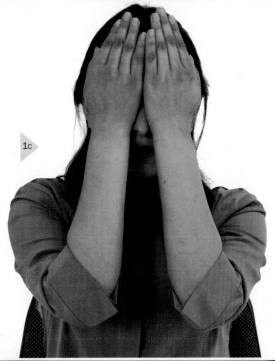

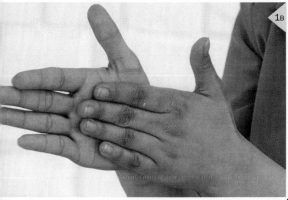

2. Blink the eyes several times as fast as possible.

DRYNESS OF THE EYES IS A COMMON COMPLAINT OF OVERWORKED AND TIRED EYES. BLINKING HELPS THE EYES TO REGAIN THEIR LOST MOISTURE. NEVER RUB ITCHY EYES.

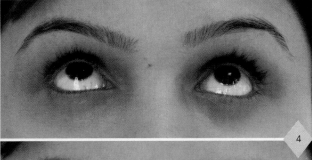

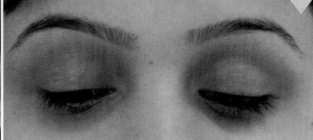

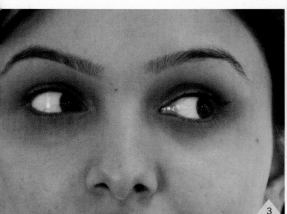

3. Keep the neck straight, and try and move the pupils of the eyes from right to left at least 8 times and left to right at least eight times.

4. Keeping the chin parallel to the floor and the neck steady, try and move the pupils up (imagine looking up at the ceiling) and down (imagine looking down at the floor). Repeat at least 8 times.

THESE EXERCISES STRENGTHEN THE MUSCLES OF THE EYES.

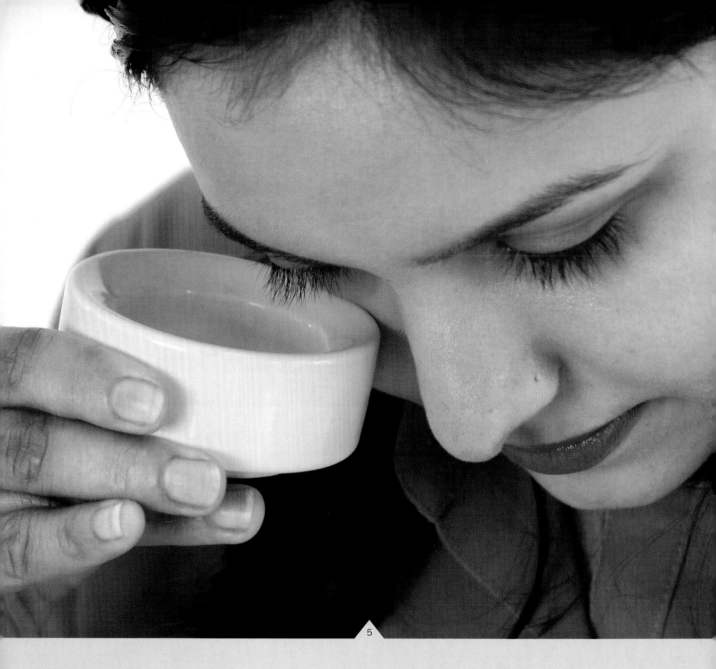

5

5. EVERY MORNING, WASH THE EYES WITH COLD, PURE DISTILLED WATER. ENSURE THAT YOUR HANDS ARE CLEAN. TAKE A CUP AND POUR SOME WATER INTO IT. PLACE ONE EYE IN THE WATER AND BLINK RAPIDLY TO CLEANSE IT. REPEAT ON THE OTHER SIDE.

Move all the time — to get water or files, or just move around to get your work done from other departments.

This constant movement will aid circulation and do away with stiff joints and the collection of blood in the lower limbs which can result in swollen feet at the end of the day.

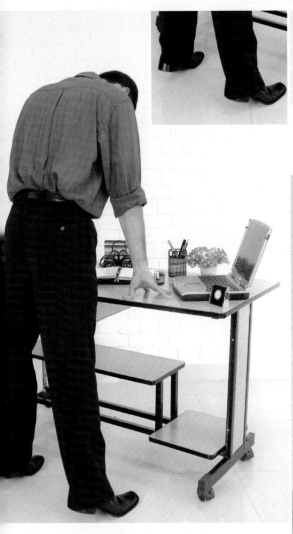

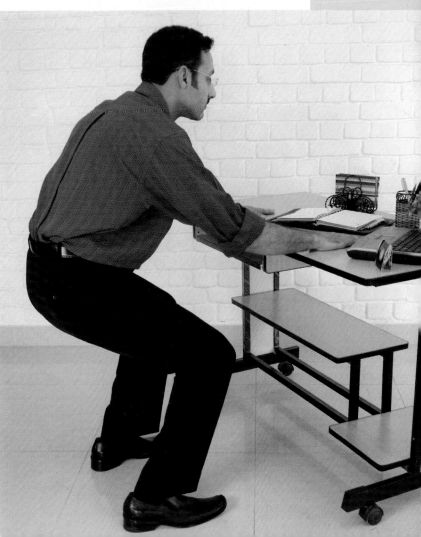

2. From the same position as in the above exercise slowly lower the hips towards the floor to simulate a sitting position. Make sure the buttocks are pushed back and down and the knees and the lower back are free of stress. Do this exercise at least 8 times a day.

This exercise strengthens the muscles of the legs and mobilises the hip joint.

Take off your shoes if the heels are too high.

1. Stand with legs at least a foot apart and place both hands on the table. Inhale and lift the heels off the floor. Exhale and rest the feet back on the floor and let the heels touch down. Repeat at least 6 times.

This exercise works the calf muscles.

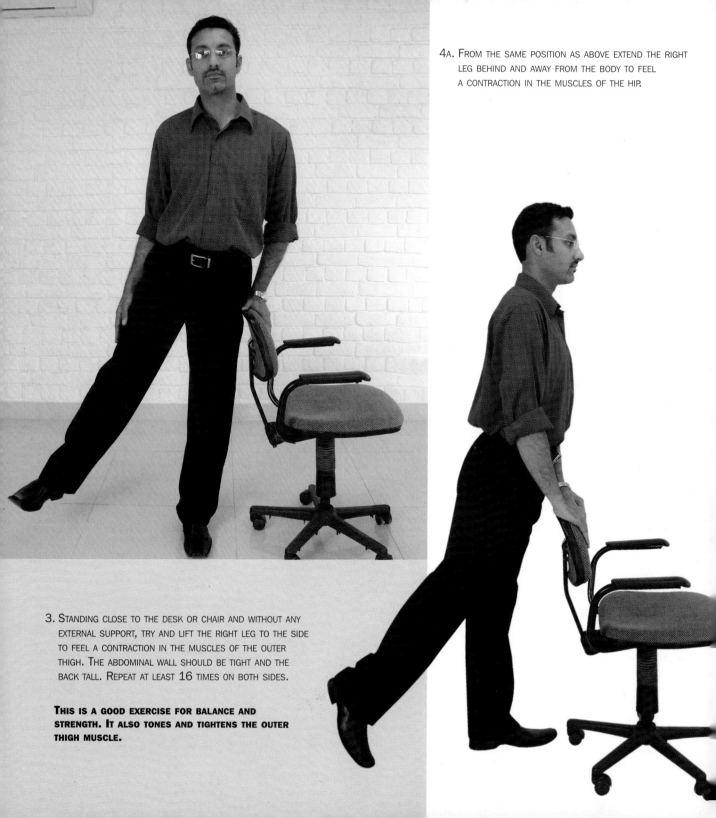

4A. FROM THE SAME POSITION AS ABOVE EXTEND THE RIGHT LEG BEHIND AND AWAY FROM THE BODY TO FEEL A CONTRACTION IN THE MUSCLES OF THE HIP.

3. STANDING CLOSE TO THE DESK OR CHAIR AND WITHOUT ANY EXTERNAL SUPPORT, TRY AND LIFT THE RIGHT LEG TO THE SIDE TO FEEL A CONTRACTION IN THE MUSCLES OF THE OUTER THIGH. THE ABDOMINAL WALL SHOULD BE TIGHT AND THE BACK TALL. REPEAT AT LEAST 16 TIMES ON BOTH SIDES.

THIS IS A GOOD EXERCISE FOR BALANCE AND STRENGTH. IT ALSO TONES AND TIGHTENS THE OUTER THIGH MUSCLE.

4B. Bring the leg to floor level and then lift the knee towards the chest. Repeat 8 to 12 times. Since it is not possible to do complete yoga postures in the office, these simple variations of the postures will be of great help.

This exercise strengthens the muscles of the hip as well as improves the flexibility of the hip joint.

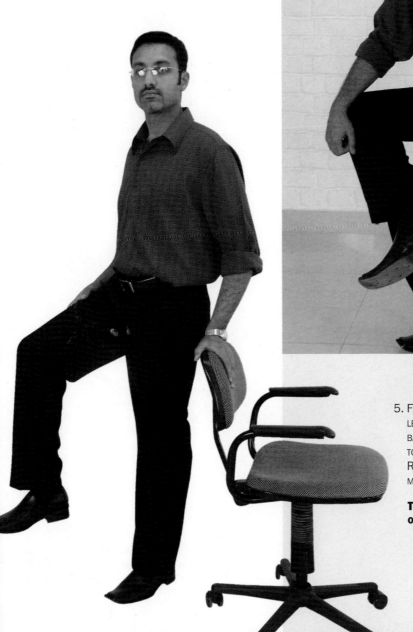

5. From the same position as above, cross the right leg over the left and simulate a sitting position by balancing on the left leg and pushing the hips towards the floor.
Repeat on the other side. Hold the stretch for one minute on either side.

This stretches the stiff muscles of the right outer thigh and the right hip.

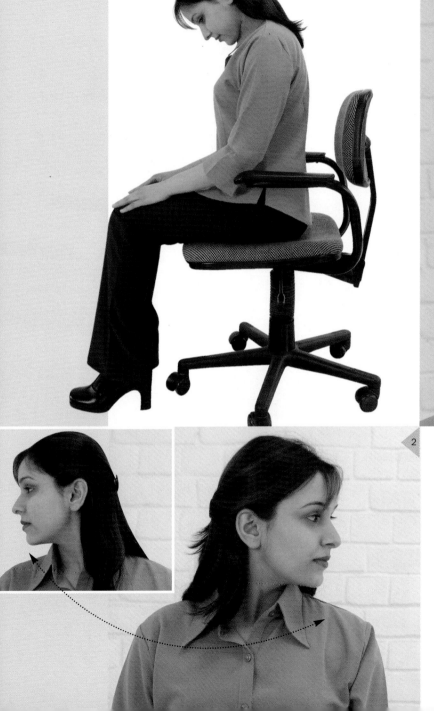

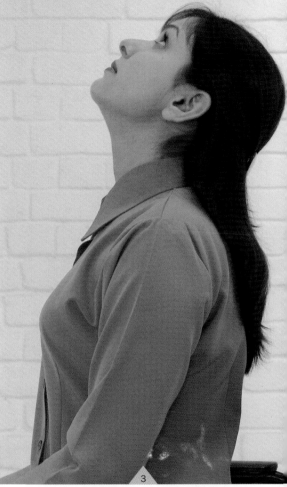

1. TO RELAX THE STRAINED MUSCLES OF THE NECK, JUST LET THE CHIN HANG TOWARDS THE CHEST AND FEEL THE STRETCH AT THE BACK OF THE NECK.
2. ROTATE THE NECK IN A FORWARD MOVEMENT ONLY. TO DO THIS FIRST TURN THE CHIN TOWARDS THE RIGHT SHOULDER AND SLOWLY MOVE IT FORWARD AND DOWN IN A SEMI-CIRCLE TOWARDS THE LEFT. GO BACK IN THE SAME SLOW MOVEMENT TOWARDS THE RIGHT AND THEN TO THE LEFT.
3. TILT THE CHIN TOWARDS THE CEILING AND HOLD.

THESE EXERCISES STRETCH AND RELAX THE MUSCLES OF THE NECK, THROAT AND UPPER BACK. REPEAT EACH EXERCISE AT LEAST 6 TIMES. HOLD FOR 10 TO 20 SECONDS IN EACH POSTURE.

SHOULDER AND ARM RELAXATION CAN BE DONE IN A SITTING OR A STANDING POSITION. THE STANDING POSITION IS PREFERRED AS IT GIVES YOU A BREAK FROM LONG HOURS OF SITTING.

1. ROTATE THE SHOULDERS FROM FRONT TO BACK AND BACK TO FRONT. REPEAT 8 TIMES.

THIS SHOULDER EXERCISE STRETCHES THE MUSCLES OF THE SHOULDERS AND THE SIDES OF THE NECK.

2A. PLACE HANDS ON THE SHOULDERS, WITH ELBOWS POINTING TO THE SIDES.

2B EXHALE AND BRING THE ELBOWS TOWARDS EACH OTHER IN FRONT OF THE BODY AS CLOSE TO EACH OTHER AS POSSIBLE.

2C. THEN LIFT BOTH ELBOWS TOWARDS THE CEILING AND BACK AND DOWN. REPEAT AT LEAST 8 TIMES.

THIS MULTIDIMENSIONAL EXERCISE STRETCHES ALL THE MUSCLES AT THE BACK OF THE SHOULDERS, THE UPPER PART OF THE SHOULDERS AND THE FRONT AND THE LOWER AREA OF THE SHOULDER JOINT, INDIVIDUALLY.

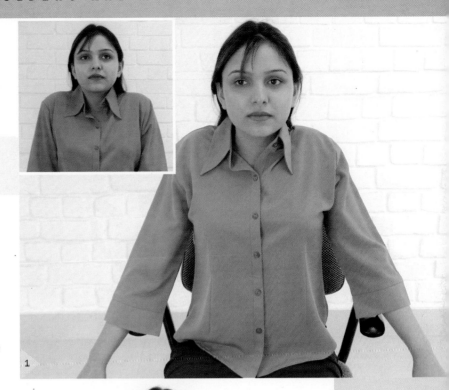

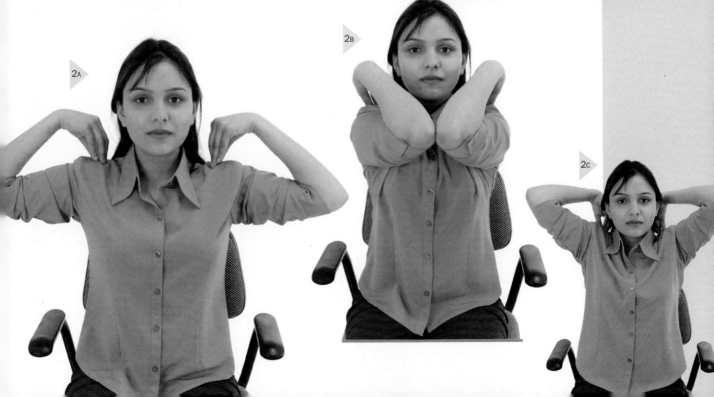

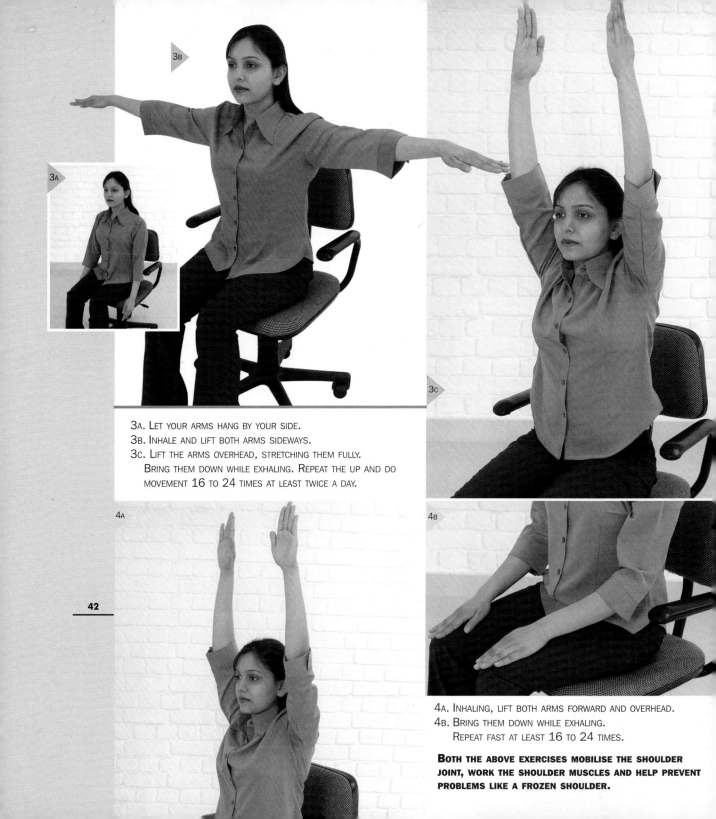

3A. LET YOUR ARMS HANG BY YOUR SIDE.

3B. INHALE AND LIFT BOTH ARMS SIDEWAYS.

3C. LIFT THE ARMS OVERHEAD, STRETCHING THEM FULLY. BRING THEM DOWN WHILE EXHALING. REPEAT THE UP AND DO MOVEMENT 16 TO 24 TIMES AT LEAST TWICE A DAY.

4A. INHALING, LIFT BOTH ARMS FORWARD AND OVERHEAD.

4B. BRING THEM DOWN WHILE EXHALING. REPEAT FAST AT LEAST 16 TO 24 TIMES.

BOTH THE ABOVE EXERCISES MOBILISE THE SHOULDER JOINT, WORK THE SHOULDER MUSCLES AND HELP PREVENT PROBLEMS LIKE A FROZEN SHOULDER.

HANDS AND FINGERS

LONG HOURS AT THE KEYBOARD CAN CAUSE PAIN AT THE BASE OF THE FINGERS AND THE KNUCKLES. STIFFNESS IN THE FINGERS AND EXTREME PAIN IN THE CARPALS AND THE METACARPALS CAN BE PREVENTED BY DOING THE FOLLOWING EXERCISES AT LEAST TWICE A DAY.

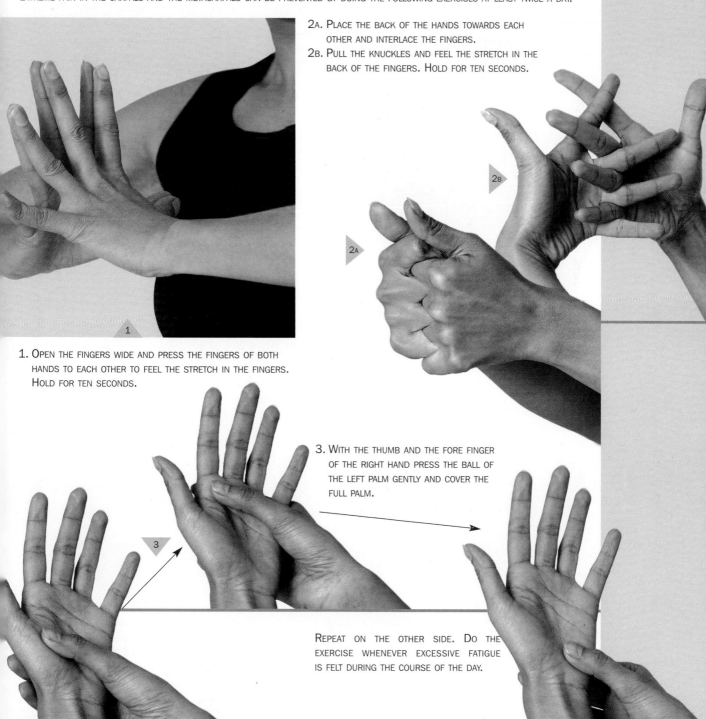

2A. PLACE THE BACK OF THE HANDS TOWARDS EACH OTHER AND INTERLACE THE FINGERS.

2B. PULL THE KNUCKLES AND FEEL THE STRETCH IN THE BACK OF THE FINGERS. HOLD FOR TEN SECONDS.

1. OPEN THE FINGERS WIDE AND PRESS THE FINGERS OF BOTH HANDS TO EACH OTHER TO FEEL THE STRETCH IN THE FINGERS. HOLD FOR TEN SECONDS.

3. WITH THE THUMB AND THE FORE FINGER OF THE RIGHT HAND PRESS THE BALL OF THE LEFT PALM GENTLY AND COVER THE FULL PALM.

REPEAT ON THE OTHER SIDE. DO THE EXERCISE WHENEVER EXCESSIVE FATIGUE IS FELT DURING THE COURSE OF THE DAY.

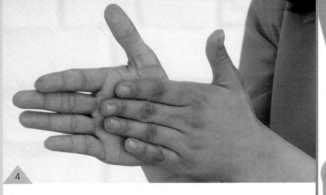

4. VIGOROUSLY RUB BOTH PALMS AGAINST EACH OTHER TO FEEL THE WARMTH IN THE PALMS.

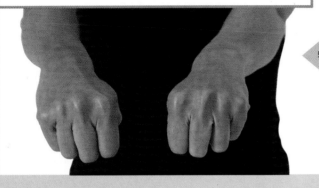

5. ROTATE THE WRISTS CLOCKWISE AND ANTICLOCKWISE TIMES. REPEAT 8 TIMES ON EACH SIDE.

DO THESE EXERCISES SEVERAL TIMES A DAY.

FEET AND ANKLES

SEDENTARY JOBS REQUIRE LITTLE OR NO MOVEMENT OF THE LOWER LIMBS WHICH RESULTS IN SWOLLEN FEET AND ANKLES, NUMBNESS IN THE TOES, ACHING OR BURNING SOLES, WEAK ANKLES AND WEAK MUSCLES OF THE FEET. INACTIVE FEET CAN LOSE THEIR STRENGTH AND FLEXIBILITY OVER A PERIOD OF TIME. INACTIVE FEET ARE ALSO VERY PRONE TO FREQUENT ACHES AND PAINS AND SUFFER PERMANENT DAMAGE DUE TO LACK OF EXERCISE. TO HELP MAINTAIN A MINIMUM LEVEL OF HEALTH IN THE FEET AND ANKLES, DO THE FOLLOWING SET OF EXERCISES AT LEAST TWICE A DAY.

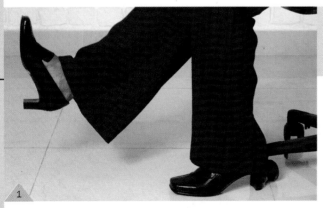

1. POINT AND FLEX THE FEET AT LEAST 8 TIMES AT FREQUENT INTERVALS DURING THE DAY.

2. ROTATE THE ANKLES CLOCKWISE AND ANTICLOCKWISE. REPEAT AT LEAST 8 TO 10 TIMES.

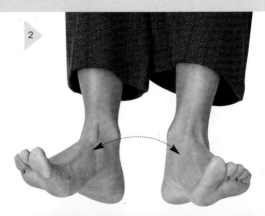

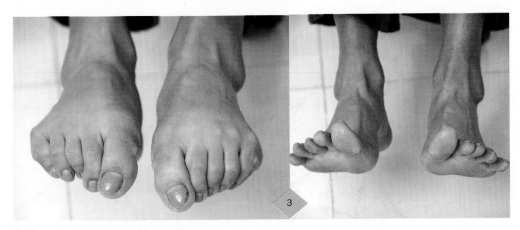

3. CURL AND EXTEND THE TOES SEVERAL TIMES.

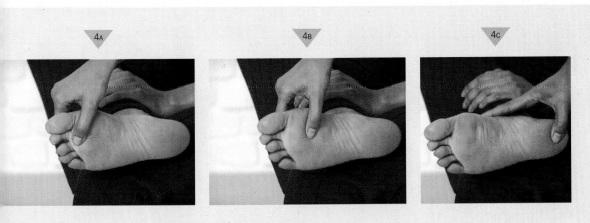

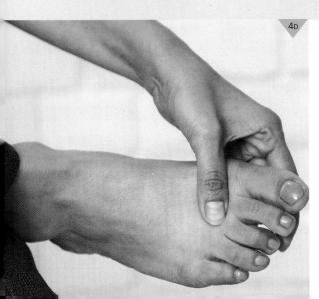

4A. TAKE OFF YOUR SHOES, PUSH BACK YOUR CHAIR AND CROSS ONE LEG OVER THE OTHER. WITH A GENTLE MOVEMENT, PRESS THE SOLE OF THE FOOT STARTING WITH THE BASE OF THE TOES.

4B. PRESS THE BALL OF THE FOOT.

4C. GO DOWN TO THE HEEL OF THE FOOT.

4D MASSAGE THE TOP OF THE FOOT AND FEEL THE HEEL AND THE FOOT RELAX.
REPEAT ON THE OTHER FOOT.

FREQUENT TRAVELLERS

People who travel frequently are envied by those who don't travel during the course of their work.
However, the picture is not as rosy as it seems. Frequent travellers have a tough time coping with travel sickness, lack of sleep, lack of exercise and jet lag.Throughout the day our waking and sleeping hours vary according the body's rhythms. These biorhythms vary in people and are influenced by various lifestyle patterns and environmental factors. These influences could be related to our professional or social life, or time and temperature changes. Some biological influences like glandular secretions also play a major role. For example **melatonin** is a hormone responsible for our sleep pattern. The production of this hormone increases with nightfall and reduces with the dawn of day. This and other natural rhythms of the body are disrupted and disturbed during long and erratic hours of travel whena flight may be at an odd hour and food is eaten late at night.

Cramped seats in aeroplanes and less leg space can take their toll on the posture and body alignment as well. The spinal column should carry the body weight and move with ease and agility, without causing stress on the upper or lower back. Incorrect posture while sitting or travelling can cause the spine to be overstressed in certain areas, thus disturbing the spinal alignment and resulting in pain and discomfort in the upper or the lower back. In extreme cases the spine gets 'locked', making it almost impossible for a person to stand upright.This could happen while:

• Standing up from a seated position • Carrying heavy bags • Standing or sitting for too long.

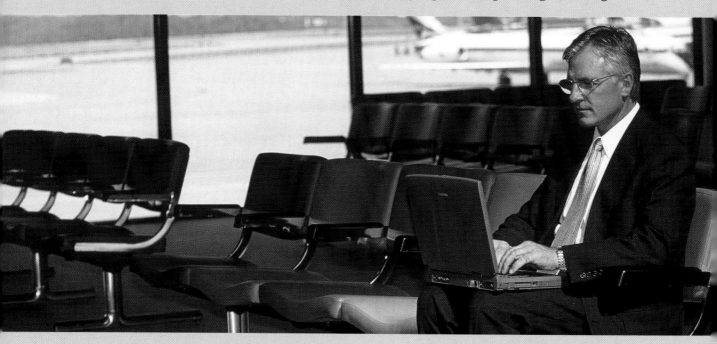

Recycled air in an aircraft, and long hours of sitting still in cramped places entail a lot of health risks like:

• Chronic fatigue • Indigestion related to disturbed eating pattern • Dehydration • Dry skin • Headaches • Stiff joints • Weak muscles • Irritability • Earache • Nausea • Backache • Postural defects like stooping shoulders
• Disturbed bowel movement - constipation or frequent motions
Lack of focus and concentration • Swollen ankles • Stress due to fear of flying

Yoga offers solutions to all these problems. The activities have to be done regularly as yoga is a way
of life and the measures should become a part of the daily routine. A few precautions associated with food and drink will ease some of the discomfort associated with long hours of travelling or frequent travelling.

Suck on a sweet as soon as the plane takes off or is about to land.

This will prevent any pressure build-up in the inner ear and the resultant pain.

Have juice and water at regular intervals to prevent dehydration.
Avoid aerated drinks as they lead to dehydration and even, mild stomach upsets.

Avoid alcohol to prevent headaches and acidity.

Eat a light diet if there is a choice, or eat before boarding but avoid greasy food.

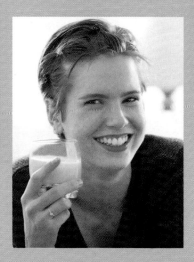

While seated, place a small pillow in the cervical region so that it supports
the spine and prevents the neck from falling side to side as you try to sleep.

Make sure the lower back rests well against the back of the chair and is fully supported
in the lumbar region. Slouching in the seat will only place unnecessary stress on the lower back.

Keep the thighs parallel to the floor and rest the feet comfortably on the floor.

Forearms should rest on the arm of the chair but not at the cost of bunching up of the shoulders.

Practice breathing exercises to avoid travel anxiety.

Carry and chew on a piece of ginger to avoid nausea.

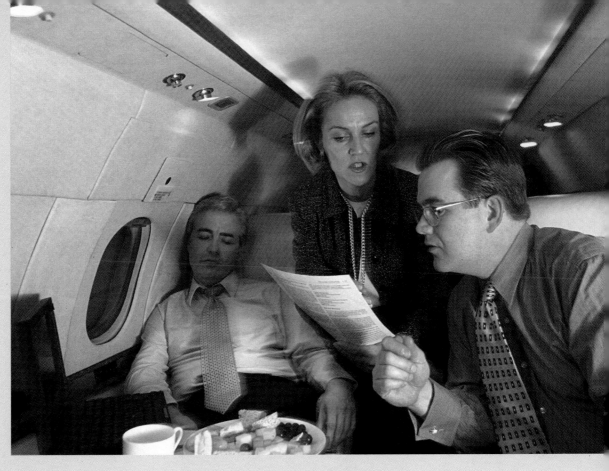

AIR TRAVEL EXERCISES

PROGRESSIVE MUSCLE RELAXATION CAN BE DONE BY FOLLOWING THE EXERCISES GIVEN BELOW.
EXERCISES DONE WHILE TRAVELLING ARE EASY TO FOLLOW, EFFECTIVE AND RESULT ORIENTED. INITIALLY, DO CONSULT THE BOOK AND THE PICTURES BUT GRADUALLY YOU WILL REMEMBER THE EXERCISES AND THEY WILL BECOME A PART OF YOUR TRAVEL LIFESTYLE. REMEMBER TO EXERCISE THE WHOLE BODY FROM NECK TO TOE AT LEAST ONCE.

1. THE NECK TAKES THE STRAIN OF LONG HOURS OF SITTING. TO RELEASE TENSION AT THE BACK OF THE NECK, PLACE THE PILLOW BELOW THE CHIN AND HOLD IT TIGHT BETWEEN THE CHIN AND THE UPPER CHEST.

   THIS WILL STRETCH THE MUSCLES AT THE BACK OF THE NECK. HOLD FOR 30 SECONDS.

2. TURN THE CHIN TOWARDS THE RIGHT SHOULDER AND TRY AND PRESS THE HEAD TO THE BACK OF THE CHAIR.

   THIS WILL STRETCH THE MUSCLES ON THE LEFT SIDE OF THE NECK. REPEAT ON THE OTHER SIDE AS WELL.

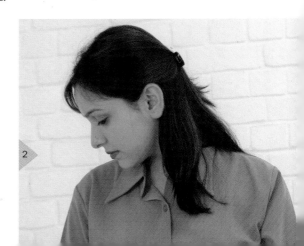

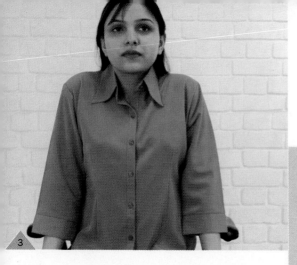

3

3. FOR THE SHOULDERS, REST BOTH HANDS AT THE SIDES. LIFT BOTH SHOULDERS TOWARDS THE EARS AND DROP THEM BACK.

4. ROTATE THE SHOULDERS, MAKING CIRCLES FORWARDS AND BACKWARDS.
REPEAT BOTH THESE EXERCISES AT LEAST 8 TIMES (SEE PAGE 11).

THESE EXERCISES WILL RELAX THE TIRED SHOULDER JOINTS AND THE MUSCLES SURROUNDING THE SHOULDER JOINTS.

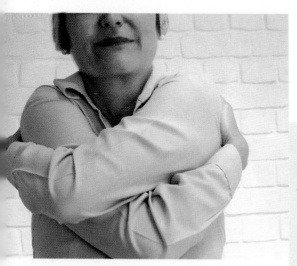

5. THE UPPER BACK GETS TIRED WITH LONG HOURS OF SITTING OR READING. CROSS THE ARMS OVER THE CHEST AND GIVE YOURSELF A GOOD HUG. HOLD THE STRETCH FOR AT LEAST 30 SECONDS.

THIS WILL STRETCH THE MUSCLES IN THE UPPER BACK.

6. FROM THE SEATED POSITION, LIFT BOTH HANDS AND HOLD THE BACK OF THE CHAIR. MOVE THE UPPER BODY AWAY FROM THE CHAIR.

THIS MOVEMENT WILL STRETCH THE FRONT OF THE TORSO FROM THE SHOULDERS TO THE CHEST AND THE WAIST.

7. PRESS CLOSED FISTS ON EITHER SIDE OF THE NAVAL (REMEMBER NOT TO COVER THE NAVAL).
INHALE AND EXPAND THE STOMACH AND BEND FORWARD WHILE EXHALING SLOWLY. THE FISTS WILL CREATE A PHYSICAL PRESSURE ON THE LOWER ABDOMINAL AREA. MAINTAIN NORMAL BREATHING WHILE HOLDING THE POSTURE.
HOLD FOR AT LEAST TEN SECONDS (SEE PAGE 79).

THIS IS A VARIATION OF A YOGIC POSTURE AND HELPS PREVENT INDIGESTION AND FLATULENCE DURING LONG HOURS OF TRAVELLING. THIS EXERCISE SHOULD BE DONE ON AN EMPTY STOMACH.

8. INHALE DEEPLY AND EXPAND THE ABDOMINAL WALL. EXHALE AND CONTRACT THE ABDOMEN TIGHT TO PULL THE NAVAL TOWARDS THE SPINE. HOLD FOR AT LEAST 10 SECONDS AND RELEASE.

THIS SEATED ABDOMINAL COMPRESSION WILL TONE AND TIGHTEN THE ABDOMINAL WALL AS WELL AS BOOST YOUR METABOLIC RATE. THIS EXERCISE IS A VARIATION OF A YOGIC POSTURE AND SHOULD BE DONE ON AN EMPTY STOMACH.

49

9. LIFT THE RIGHT KNEE, HOLD WITH BOTH HANDS AND PULL IT TOWARDS THE CHEST. THE SEAT SHOULD BE UPRIGHT AND THE SEAT BELT LOOSE WHILE PERFORMING THIS EXERCISE. HOLD THE STRETCH FOR AT LEAST 10 SECONDS. REPEAT TWO TO THREE TIMES ON EACH SIDE.

THIS WILL RELEASE ANY SORENESS IN THE BUTTOCKS AND MOBILISE THE HIP JOINT. REPEAT WHENEVER THE LOWER BODY FEELS TIRED, INACTIVE AND HEAVY.

10. STRETCH BOTH LEGS FAR FORWARD BELOW THE SEAT IN FRONT AND LIFT THE WHOLE BODY UP AND AWAY FROM THE CHAIR IN A SLANTING POSITION. THE SHOULDERS AND THE ARMS SHOULD SUPPORT THE BODY AND THE FEET SHOULD ANCHOR IT TO THE FLOOR. HOLD FOR 10 SECONDS AND RELEASE.

THIS WILL STRETCH THE ABDOMINAL AREA AND HELP STRAIGHTEN THE SPINE, GIVING IT SOME RELIEF FROM LONG HOURS OF SITTING. THIS CAN BE DONE OFTEN DURING A LONG FLIGHT.

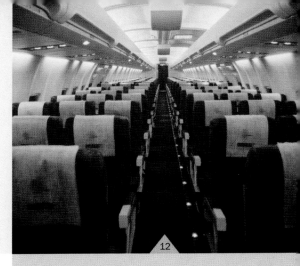

12.

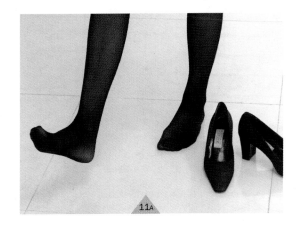

11A.

11A. REMOVE YOUR SHOES AND POINT AND FLEX YOUR FEET SEVERAL TIMES.

11B. ROTATE THE ANKLES CLOCKWISE AND ANTICLOCKWISE SEVERAL TIMES TOO.

THIS SIMPLE EXERCISE WILL PREVENT POOLING OF THE BLOOD IN THE LOWER LIMBS AND WILL, IN TURN, PREVENT SWELLING OF THE FEET, AS WELL AS PAIN AND BURNING IN THE SOLES OF THE FEET.

12. WHENEVER THE BODY FEELS EXTREMELY TIRED, AND IT IS SAFE TO STAND UP, WALK IN THE AISLE FOR A FEW MINUTES OR JUST STAND IN FRONT OF THE CHAIR AND RAISE BOTH ARMS TOWARDS THE CEILING WHILE INHALING.
- EXHALE AND BRING THE ARMS DOWN BY THE SIDE. REPEAT AT LEAST 3 TIMES.

13. LATE NIGHT FLIGHTS, AN ERRATIC SLEEP PATTERN AND LONG HOURS OF TRAVELLING RESULT IN A CHRONIC FEELING OF FATIGUE AND CAN BE AN UNDERLYING CAUSE OF HEADACHES. TRY AND SIT WITH THE EYES CLOSED EVEN IF SLEEP EVADES YOU. THE NECK AND SHOULDER MUSCLES SHOULD BE RELAXED AND SUPPORTED WITH THE SMALL PILLOW. REST THE HANDS IN THE LAP AND PRACTISE ABDOMINAL BREATHING.
- INHALE AND EXPAND THE CHEST AND STOMACH. TAKE FOUR TO SIX SECONDS TO DO THIS.
- EXHALE AND RELAX THE WHOLE BODY AND TAKE AS LONG AS POSSIBLE TO ACHIEVE A LONG AND SLOW EXPIRATION. TRY AND INHALE AND EXHALE THROUGH THE NOSE UNLESS THE NOSE IS BLOCKED DUE TO A COLD.

THIS EXERCISE WILL RELAX YOUR TIRED BODY AND MIND. IT WILL EASE MUSCULAR AND MENTAL TENSION, AND GET RID OF A HEADACHE CAUSED BY TENSION, ANXIETY OR INDIGESTION. THIS BREATHING SHOULD SPECIALLY BE DONE BY PEOPLE WHO SUFFER FROM FEAR OF FLYING, AND THEY SHOULD DO THIS AT THE TIME OF TAKE OFF AND LANDING.

Fight jet lag the moment you step off the plane.

Go outdoors and absorb the natural light of day.

Exercise for at least half an hour but keep it light and simple as there may be a bit
of disorientation left over from a jet lag. A medium-paced walk will do.

Stay awake and go to sleep only at the local sleep time. In order to do this,
try the auto-suggestion yoga technique given below.

YOGA RELAXATION THROUGH AUTO-SUGGESTION

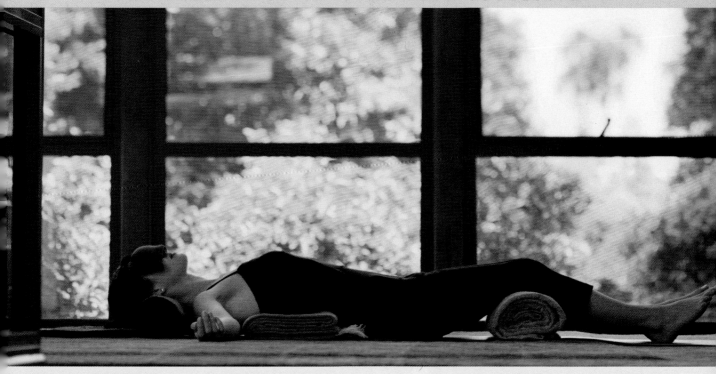

- LIE DOWN ON THE BACK WITH BOTH LEGS SLIGHTLY APART.
- MAINTAIN DEEP ABDOMINAL BREATHING THROUGHOUT. FEEL THE ABDOMINAL WALL EXPAND WHILE INHALING AND RELAX WHILE EXHALING. THE WHOLE BODY SHOULD FEEL HEAVY AND RELAXED WHILE EXHALING.
- MENTALLY FOCUS ON THE FEET AND THE ANKLES. IMAGINE THE STRESS AND PAIN GOING OUT OF THE BODY WITH EVERY EXHALATION. TRAVEL UP FROM THE FEET TO THE SHINS, THE CALVES, KNEES, FRONT OF THE THIGHS AND THE BACK OF THE THIGHS, THE HIP AND LOWER BACK, THE MIDDLE BACK AND THE TORSO, THE CHEST AND THE UPPER BACK, FINALLY THE NECK, SHOULDERS, ARMS, AND PALMS AND FINGERS.
- REPEAT THE PROCESS FROM HEAD TO FOOT.

Note. Light music helps one relax while performing this technique.

A HEALTHY DIET PLAN

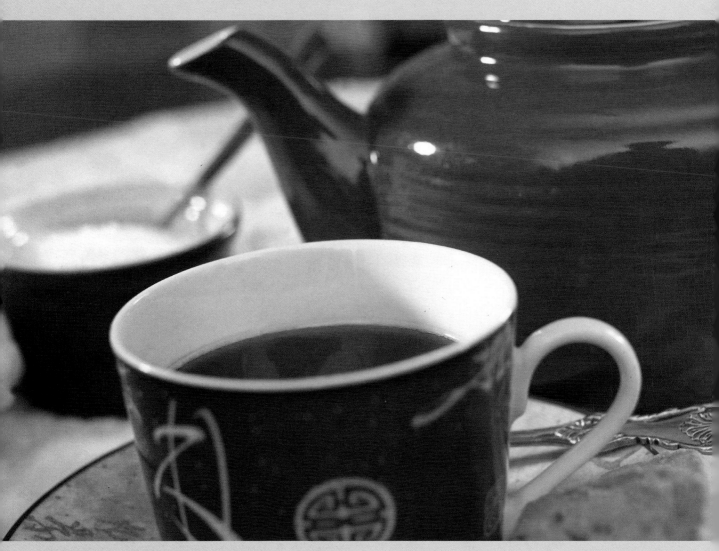

**All the advice given here is for people with no chronic ailments.
It is advisable to undergo a medical check-up before following these suggestions.**

Counting calories can be quite a task, especially if you wish to shed excess fat. Such desperate measures seldom have to be taken if you follow an easy diet plan which provides the essential nutrients from easily available food items. A moderate diet not only appeases hunger; it provides nourishment and energy to cope with day-to-day activities.

SIMPLE DOS AND DON'TS

1. Never ignore hunger.

2. Eat frequent but small meals rather than one large meal.

3. Snack only on fruits and salads.

4. Restrict yourself to only one helping of cereal a day.

5. Avoid fasting and food deprivation as this will merely lead to binging, acidity, irritability and raise your stress level.

6. Opt for low fat and low sugar foods whenever possible.

7. Avoid processed foods and aerated drinks. Drink alcohol in moderation.

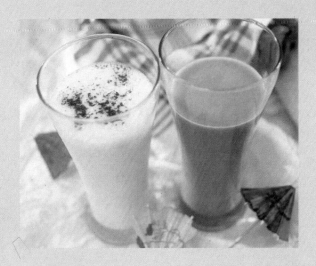

8. Eat in moderation and stay away from a second helping.

9. Eat an early dinner and eat a light meal.

10. Make breakfast and lunch your main meals.

11. Restrict yourself to one cup of tea or coffee during working hours.
Have juice instead, and drink at least 8 to 10 glasses of water every day.

12. Smoking should be a big No-No.

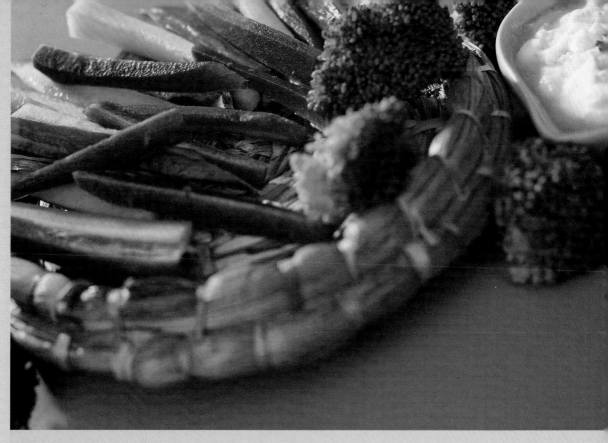

AN EASY-TO-FOLLOW DIET PLAN

Early morning
- Two glasses of lukewarm water or a cup of tea with less sugar (no sugar for those who wish to lose weight)
- One/two low fat and low sugar biscuits

Breakfast
- One small bowl of cereal (oats or broken wheat) with skimmed milk
- One helping of fruit

OR
- One boiled egg with one toast (brown bread)
- One helping of fruit

OR
- One oil-free paratha (stuffed with lentils or cottage cheese)
- A bowl of fat-free yogurt

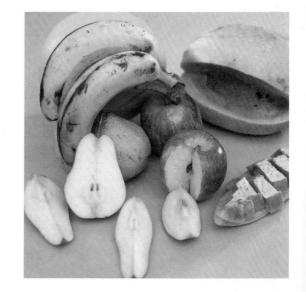

Mid-Morning
• One helping of fruit OR one glass of skimmed milk

Lunch
• Two slices of brown bread / two small chapattis
• One helping of non-vegetarian food
  (avoid red meat)/ one small bowl of dal
• A bowl of yogurt
• Two helpings of vegetables
• A large helping of salad with an oil-free dressing

Evening Snack
Tea / coffee with two low fat biscuits
OR A low fat vegetable sandwich

Dinner
Dinner can be almost the same as lunch

But for weight watchers
• A bowl of soup
• A tofu salad
OR
• A bowl of soup
• A small portion of grilled fish or chicken
• Salad with a low fat dressing

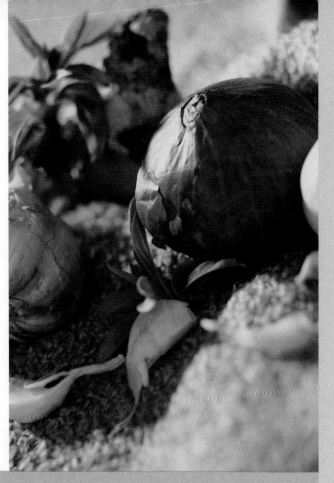

USEFUL TIPS

• Use oil sparingly.
• To appease a sweet tooth, have two dates or a piece of jaggery. Avoid sugary foods.
• Eat non-fried rice and potatoes in moderation.
• If under stress, avoid highly spiced food, and excessive intake of tea and coffee.
• Green tea is an excellent stress buster and can be had at regular intervals through the working day. Camomile, jasmine, mint and lemon are great flavours.
• Consume less animal proteins as they have a tendency to increase acid production in the body.
• When under stress, immunity is drastically reduced. Eating foods rich in vitamins, minerals and flavnoids will keep the immunity levels high. Fresh fruits and vegetables will also be beneficial.
• Avoid processed foods.
• Those trying to lose weight should avoid fad diets / difficult diets as they are difficult to follow in the long run.
• Just cutting down on one small drink a day and including one hour of exercise each day will help burn calories faster and control weight better.

STRESS BUSTERS:
YOGIC BREATHING

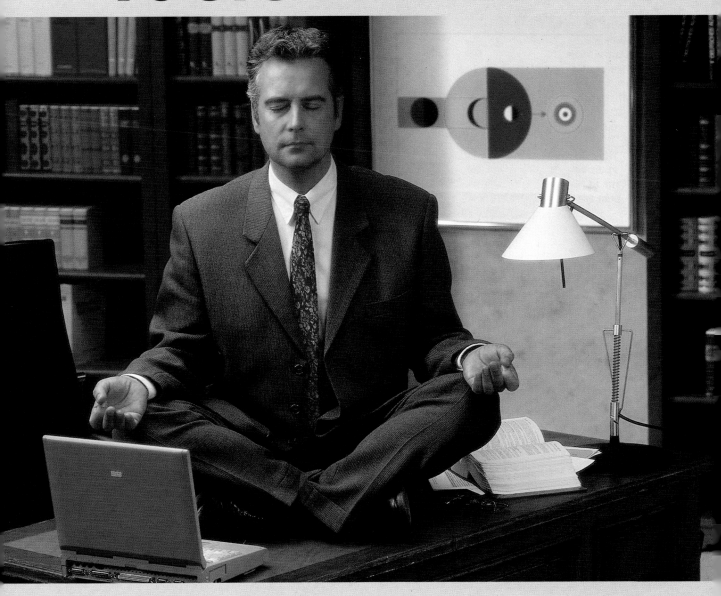

Fitness and health is in our own hands and we can all prepare ourselves physically and mentally to handle stress at work and in our personal life. The regular practice of yogic breathing not only calms the nerves but also brings the autonomous nervous system(the involuntary system) under control. Yoga breathing exercises provide a complete mind-body-soul workout.

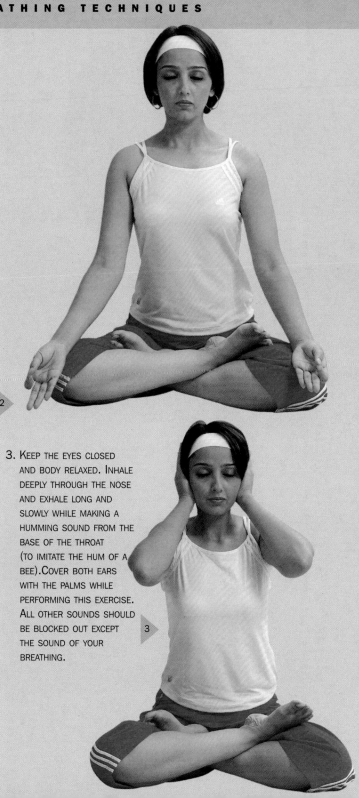

1. SIT WITH THE BACK STRAIGHT. IF YOU CANNOT SIT CROSS-LEGGED IN THE LOTUS POSTURE (SEE PAGE 92) ON THE FLOOR OR IN *VAJRASANA* (SEE PAGE 78), THEN SIT IN A STRAIGHT-BACKED CHAIR.

- PLACE BOTH HANDS ON THE THIGHS AND TAKE IN LONG DEEP BREATHS IN THROUGH THE NOSTRILS AND EXHALE THROUGH THE NOSTRILS AS WELL. THE CHEST AND ABDOMEN SHOULD EXPAND WHILE INHALING, AND CONTRACT WHILE EXHALING. REPEAT FOR A MINUTE OR TWO TO START WITH AND PROGRESS TO THREE ROUNDS OF ONE MINUTE EACH AS THE BREATHING CAPACITY IMPROVES.

MOST PEOPLE DO NOT BREATHE CORRECTLY AND THIS EXERCISE WILL TRAIN ONE TO FOLLOW THE CORRECT RHYTHMIC PATTERN OF BREATHING. ONCE THIS SIMPLE TECHNIQUE HAS BEEN MASTERED ADD ON THE FOLLOWING BREATHING EXERCISES AS WELL.

NOTE. IN THE BEGINNING IT IS A GOOD IDEA TO PLACE BOTH PALMS ON YOUR ABDOMEN TO FEEL THE MOVEMENT OF THE ABDOMINAL WALL WITH EACH BREATH.

2. REPEAT THE SAME EXERCISE AS THE ONE GIVEN ABOVE BUT TRY AND INHALE AND EXHALE MORE FORCEFULLY AND QUICKLY. WHILE DOING THIS THE BREATH WILL BECOME SHORTER AND FASTER. THE ABDOMINAL WALL SHOULD MOVE IN AND OUT FAST AND WITH FORCE (LIKE BELLOWS).

- AFTER A MINUTE, RETURN TO NORMAL BREATHING.
- FINALLY, FOLLOW WITH THE SLOW BREATHING RECOMMENDED EARLIER.

3. KEEP THE EYES CLOSED AND BODY RELAXED. INHALE DEEPLY THROUGH THE NOSE AND EXHALE LONG AND SLOWLY WHILE MAKING A HUMMING SOUND FROM THE BASE OF THE THROAT (TO IMITATE THE HUM OF A BEE).COVER BOTH EARS WITH THE PALMS WHILE PERFORMING THIS EXERCISE. ALL OTHER SOUNDS SHOULD BE BLOCKED OUT EXCEPT THE SOUND OF YOUR BREATHING.

IN THE BEGINNING THESE EXERCISES CAN MAKE YOU DIZZY BUT WITH PRACTICE, THEY WILL BE EASY TO DO FOR A LONGER PERIOD OF TIME. BOTH PATTERNS 1 AND 2 SHOULD TAKE AT LEAST 7 TO 8 MINUTES EACH.

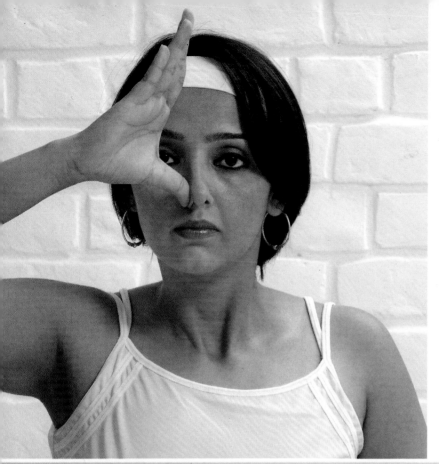

4. ALTERNATE NOSTRIL BREATHING: WITH THE THUMB OF THE RIGHT HAND CLOSE THE RIGHT NOSTRIL AND INHALE THROUGH THE LEFT.
- CLOSE THE LEFT NOSTRIL AND HOLD THE BREATH IN FOR A FEW SECONDS.
- OPEN THE RIGHT NOSTRIL AND EXHALE LONG AND SLOW THROUGH THE RIGHT NOSTRIL.
- NEXT INHALE FROM THE RIGHT AND EXHALE FROM THE LEFT. REPEAT THIS ALTERNATE FORM OF BREATHING FOR AS LONG AS POSSIBLE (UP TO 5 MINUTES).

NOTE. USE ONLY THE THUMB AND THE RING FINGER OF THE RIGHT HAND TO PERFORM THIS BREATHING EXERCISE.

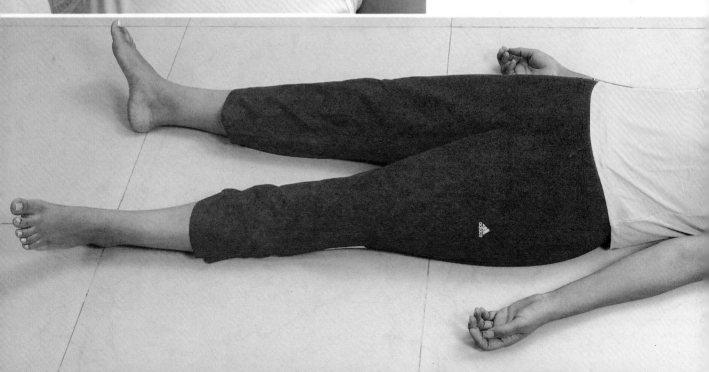

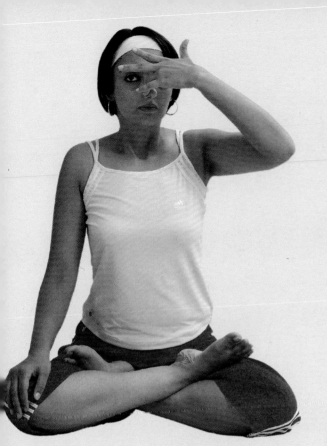

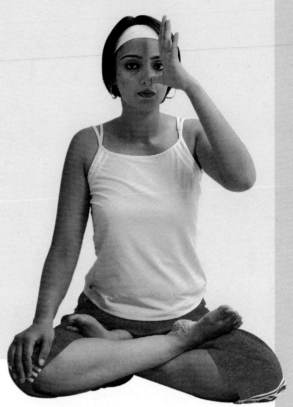

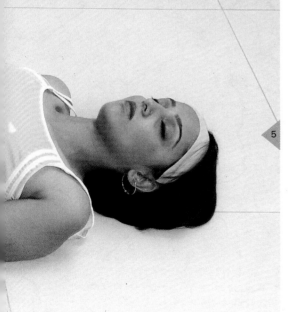

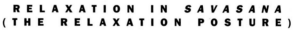

5

RELAXATION IN *SAVASANA* (THE RELAXATION POSTURE)

5. *SAVASANA* IS ADVISED WHENEVER FATIGUE SETS IN. ANY FORM OF YOGA IS BEST DONE WHEN THE MIND AS WELL AS THE BODY ARE RELAXED AND FREE OF TENSION.

• LIE DOWN ON THE BACK AND KEEP THE WHOLE BODY LOOSE AND RELAXED. FOCUS ON EACH BREATH AS IT GOES IN AND OUT. THE BODY WILL LEARN TO RELAX WITH EACH EXHALATION AND IN A FEW WEEKS YOU WILL MASTER THE ART OF TOTAL RELAXATION.

CAUTION. NEVER DO BREATHING EXERCISES SOON AFTER A MEAL.

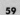

REJUVENATING EFFECTS OF MEDITATION

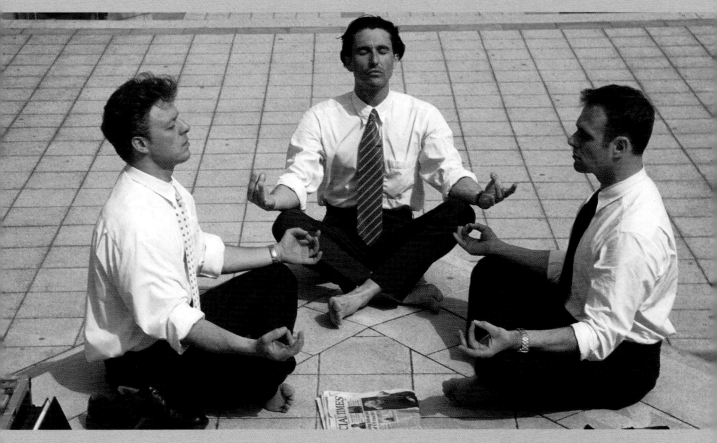

Meditation has proven to be successful in all kinds of situations when there is physical or mental stress. Life today certainly demands de-stressing in any manner possible. Though it is difficult to define the technique which is best for every individual, the techniques given below are well tested and easy to follow. Even five minutes of meditation, to start with, can provide immense benefit. It is said that twenty minutes of meditation is as rejuvenating as eight hours of sleep. Regular practice of meditation reduces instances of stress-related diseases like respiratory ailments, hypertension, skin ailments, insomnia, irritability, and dependence on alcohol and tobacco.

To begin with, sit in a posture most comfortable to you. The ideal is, of course, the Lotus Posture or *Padmasana* (see page 92) or *Vajrasana* (see page 78). If sitting on the floor is difficult, sit on a straight-backed chair. The spine must be in a neutral position with no slouching or hyper-extending. The neck and shoulders must be relaxed.

TECHNIQUE 1

SELECT AN IMAGE AND STUDY IT CAREFULLY BEFORE STARTING. CLOSE YOUR EYES AND SIT STILL. BRING THE IMAGE INTO FOCUS AND FILL IN EACH MINUTE DETAIL AS YOU SAW IT. TRY AND CHOOSE A PLEASANT, STRESS-FREE PICTURE LIKE A SEASHORE OR A GARDEN OR THE PICTURE OF A LOVED ONE.

TECHNIQUE 2

REPEAT A MANTRA OVER AND OVER AGAIN FOR THE TIME THAT YOU KEEP FOR THE MEDITATION.

TECHNIQUE 3

COUNT FROM NUMBERS ONE TO TEN OVER AND OVER AGAIN. REPEAT THESE NUMBERS SILENTLY TO YOURSELF.

TECHNIQUE 4

IN A DARK ROOM LIGHT A CANDLE OR IDENTIFY A SPOT ON A WHITE WALL. FOCUS ON IT AS A MEDITATION TECHNIQUE.

MEDITATION STILLS THE RESTLESS MIND. IT DOES NOT NUMB THE MIND BUT MAKES IT AWARE AND ALIVE. EXTERNAL THOUGHTS AND DISTURBANCES LIKE SOUNDS, SMELLS AND LIGHT MAY CAUSE ANNOYANCE BUT THE TRICK IS TO BE AN UNAFFECTED OBSERVER TO ALL THAT PASSES EXTERNALLY AND INTERNALLY. PLEASANT OR UNPLEASANT THOUGHTS AND DESIRES THAT MAY OR MAY NOT HAVE BEEN FULFILLED, PEOPLE AND THOUGHTS ASSOCIATED WITH PEOPLE AND INCIDENTS DEFINITELY BREAK INTO YOUR THOUGHTS WHILE MEDITATING. DO NOT ESCAPE THESE INTERFERENCES BUT JUST BE AN OBSERVER TO ALL THAT IS GOING ON, AND THE MOMENT YOU REALISE THAT YOUR MIND HAS SHIFTED FROM MEDITATION TO SOMETHING ELSE, GENTLY BRING IT BACK INTO FOCUS WITHOUT STRESS OR IRRITABILITY OR ANY SENSE OF FRUSTRATION. WITH REGULAR PRACTICE, THE INCIDENTS OF MENTAL STRAYING WILL REDUCE AND A PERMANENT CALM WILL PENETRATE YOUR BEING. EVEN IF OTHER THOUGHTS DO INTERFERE WITH YOUR MEDITATION, THE QUALITY OF THE THOUGHTS WILL BECOME LESS STRESSFUL AND MORE CALMING IN NATURE.

WORKOUT PLANS

Once you become regular with the yogic exercises at your workplace and reap the benefits of these simple but effective methods of keeping fit, you will undoubtedly feel like exploring the benefits of yoga even more. This section of the book serves this purpose. Long workout schedules are impossible for people hard pressed for time but twenty to thirty minutes is all that is needed to maintain a basic level of fitness in an individual. This fitness routine may not aid in drastic weight reduction or vigorous bodybuilding but will certainly help you to stay agile and cope with the functional stress the body is put through while coping with daily work schedules, and reduce mental stress as well.

A good start to the program would be to get up a half hour earlier than usual and adopt the programme. Fitness routines done early in the day set a kind of a pattern where discipline becomes a way of life and fitness becomes a lifestyle change rather than a chore.

A basic medical check-up is advisable. Have enough water preferably after the workout.

Kit out in suitable clothes for the exercise programme.

WORKOUT 1: 22 MINUTES

WARM-UP: 7 MINUTES
1. REFER TO THE LIMBERING UP EXERCISES (SEE PAGES 65-70), AND SELECT ONE EXERCISE FROM EACH SECTION.
2. WALK ON THE SPOT FOR 2 MINUTES TO REMOVE STIFFNESS FROM THE JOINTS AND MUSCLES. MOVE ELBOWS BY YOUR SIDE AS YOU WALK.

MAIN ACTIVITY: 10 MINUTES
1. TWELVE SUN SALUTATIONS OR *SURYANAMASKARS* (SEE PAGES 95-96).
2. TWO SUPINE AND 2 PRONE POSTURES (ASANAS) FOR THE ABDOMEN AND THE BACK, RESPECTIVELY:
   A. *UTTANPADASANA* (SEE PAGE 86).
   B. *NAVASANA* (SEE PAGE 87).
   C. *DHANURASANA* (SEE PAGE 91).
   D. *SALBHASANA* (SEE PAGE 90).

BREATHING EXERCISES: 2 MINUTES (SEE PAGES 56-59).

SAVASANA: 3 MINUTES (SEE PAGE 59).

WORKOUT 2: 20 MINUTES

THIS IS EXCELLENT FOR FREQUENT TRAVELLERS.
1. WALKING OUTDOORS: 10 MINUTES
2. SIX SUN SALUTATIONS OR *SURYANAMASKARS* (SEE PAGES 95-96): 8 MINUTES
3. SLEEPING POSE OR *SAVASANA* (SEE PAGE 59): 2 MINUTES

WORKOUT 3: 30 MINUTES (WITH PROGRESSION UP TO 1 HOUR AFTER 16 WEEKS AS GIVEN IN THE WORKOUT PROGRESSIONS BELOW)

PEOPLE WITH ENOUGH TIME SHOULD ADOPT THIS METHOD.

WORKOUT 3 - WEEK 1 TO WEEK 4: AT LEAST 30 MINUTES

1. FOCUS ON ALL THE LIMBERING UP EXERCISES (SEE PAGES 65-70).
2. FOLLOW THIS UP WITH THE STANDING AND BALANCING POSTURES (SEE PAGES 75-78).

NOTE. OBESE PEOPLE NEED TO ADD A WALK OR A SWIM TO LOSE EXCESS WEIGHT FASTER AND GO ON A LOW FAT, LOW SUGAR DIET IN ADDITION TO DOING THE EXERCISES.

WORKOUT 3 - WEEK 5 TO WEEK 8: 40 MINUTES

AS FLEXIBILITY INCREASES, ADD ON TWO SITTING POSTURES (SEE PAGES 78 TO 84) EVERY ALTERNATE DAY TILL ALL THE SITTING POSTURES ARE INCLUDED.

WORKOUT 3 - WEEK 9 TO WEEK 12: 45 MINUTES

1. ALL THE LIMBERING UP EXERCISES (SEE PAGES 65-70).
2. SIX SUN SALUTATIONS OR *SURYANAMASKARS* (SEE PAGES 95-96).
3. ALL THE BALANCING POSTURES (SEE PAGES 77-78).
4. ALL THE SITTING POSTURES (SEE PAGES 78-84).

WORKOUT 3 - WEEK 13 TO 16: 1 HOUR

1. ALL THE LIMBERING UP EXERCISES (SEE PAGES 65-70).
3. SIX SUN SALUTATIONS OR *SURYANAMASKARS* (SEE PAGES 95-96).
4. ALL THE BALANCING POSTURES (SEE PAGES 77-78).
5. SIX SITTING POSITIONS (SEE PAGES 78-84).
6. ALL PRONE POSTURES (SEE PAGES 89-91).
ALL THE SUPINE POSTURES (SEE PAGES 85-89).

NOTE. BREATHING EXERCISES CAN BE DONE AFTER PERFORMING THE POSTURES AND ALWAYS FINISH WITH THE LYING POSE OR *SAVASANA* FOR TWO MINUTES.

THE FINAL STAGE OF THE WORKOUT 3 PLAN SHOULD INCLUDE POSTURES/*ASANAS* FROM ALL SECTIONS. DIFFERENT *ASANAS* SHOULD BE DONE EACH WEEK TO COVER ALL THE POSTURES IN THE BOOK. THE MORE DIFFICULT ONES LIKE THE LOTUS POSTURE, *PADMASANA*, AND THE SHOULDER STAND, *SARVANGASANA*, NEED CONSTANT PRACTICE AND SHOULD BE INCLUDED IN EACH EXERCISE SESSION AFTER WEEK 8.
ONLY WITH REGULAR PRACTICE WILL YOU ACCRUE THE BENEFITS OF ALL THE YOGA POSTURES, BREATHING EXERCISES AND RELAXATION.

THE ESSENCE OF YOGA

Yoga means union — union with nature, with your inner self and with the universal energy.
It is a way of life that shows a path towards a peaceful, healthy and complete existence.
It is a mind, body and soul workout which is well suited for the healthy and not so healthy, and benefits individuals of all age groups. It is not just an exercise program. The unique feature of yoga is its curative properties. The postures or *asanas*, the cleansing processes or *kriyas* and *bandas*, the breath control or *pranayama*, and exercises have a beneficial effect on the mind, body and soul. All these put together and done in a correct order bring the autonomous system under regulation, thereby reducing occasions of illness, reducing severity of diseases and, in some cases, curing the diseases completely.

The eightfold path of YOGA comprises:
1. *Yama* — Determination, 2. *Niyama* — Discipline, 3. *Asanas* — Postures, 4. *Pranayama* — Breath control
5. *Pratyahara* — Being centred, 6. *Dharana* — Concentration, 7. *Dhyana* — Meditation
8. *Samadhi* — Self-realisation

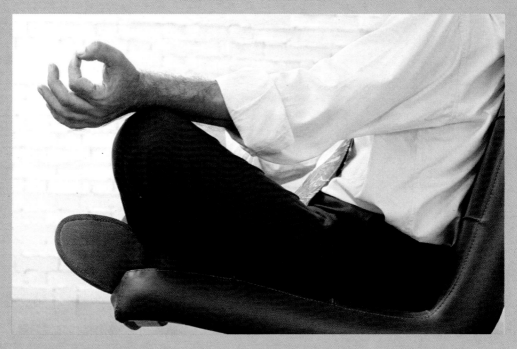

The first three bring peace and harmony at a physical level, cure ailments,
and increase concentration and determination in an individual.
Pranayama and *Pratyahara* teach the art of breath control and, thereby,
equip you to control your mind, thoughts and actions.
The last three are the stages of yoga that take you along the path
of self-realisation and spiritual evolvement.
However it is the combination of all the eight disciplines that actually
takes you to the state of good health and well-being.

THE NATURE OF *YOGASANAS*

There are close to 84,00,000 yogic postures, *yogasanas*, and most of them are derived from nature itself.
A number of postures imitate beings of the animal world like the tortoise and the hare,
while others imitate inanimate objects like mountains and boats. Plants, trees and flowers have their own place as well.

It is not how many postures or *asanas* you can do but how well you can execute them that matters.
Yoga is more about the perfection of being centred and focused, and being a challenge only to yourself.
Each posture should be performed with complete concentration and self-control. The breathing pattern should be regulated
according to the posture and the progress has to be systematic and slow.

GETTING STARTED

As with any exercise program, a warm-up before the workout is absolutely essential. Performing *yogasanas*
without limbering up can lead to injuries. Slow and systematic progress is advised and a series of warm-up exercises is to be followed
for complete mobilisation and lubrication of joints, to increase the core temperature of your body and remove muscular viscosity.

Yoga should be performed on an empty stomach. No food or water should be ingested two to four hours prior to the workout
and during the workout itself. Dress in light and comfortable loose clothing to perform the *asanas* with ease. There is no requirement
of any kind of footwear to do a yoga session. All you need is a yoga mat which could made of any non-slip fibre and has very light
cushioning. Perform all the *yogasanas* facing the east if possible. To obtain the best results they should be done early in the
morning before the working day begins. However, people with time constraints can do the exercises in the evening as well.

LIMBERING UP

Stand with both feet together, arms by your side and neck and shoulder muscles relaxed. Keep the abdominal muscles tight
and thighs pressed together. Try and perform each exercise without any jerks, but at the same time stretch the muscles and
ligaments to loosen the joints and warm up the body. Breathing should be normal during all the exercises.
Repeat each exercise at least eight times and hold each posture for 10 to 30 seconds.

1. Side to side

TURN YOUR CHIN TOWARDS THE RIGHT SHOULDER AND THEN TOWARDS THE LEFT. FEEL THE PULL IN THE MUSCLES OF THE NECK.

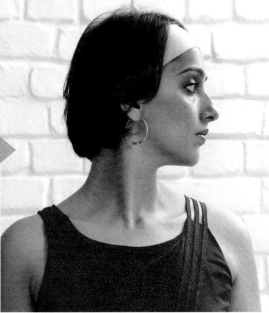

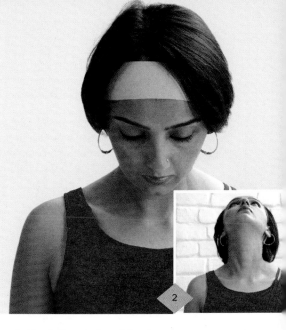

2. Neck forward and back

TAKE YOUR CHIN DOWN SO THAT IT TOUCHES THE CHEST AND YOU FEEL A PULL AT THE BACK OF THE NECK.
NEXT, TAKE THE NECK BACK SO THE CHIN IS POINTING TOWARD THE CEILING AND YOU FEEL A STRETCH IN THE THROAT.

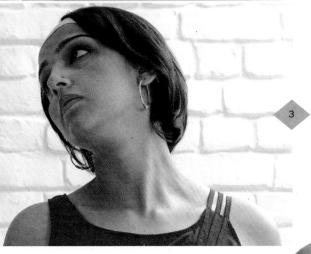

3. Forward neck rotations

POSITION THE CHIN IN THE DIRECTION OF THE RIGHT SHOULDER. MOVE IN A FORWARD AND DOWN MOVEMENT TOWARDS THE LEFT SHOULDER AND THEN BACK AGAIN.

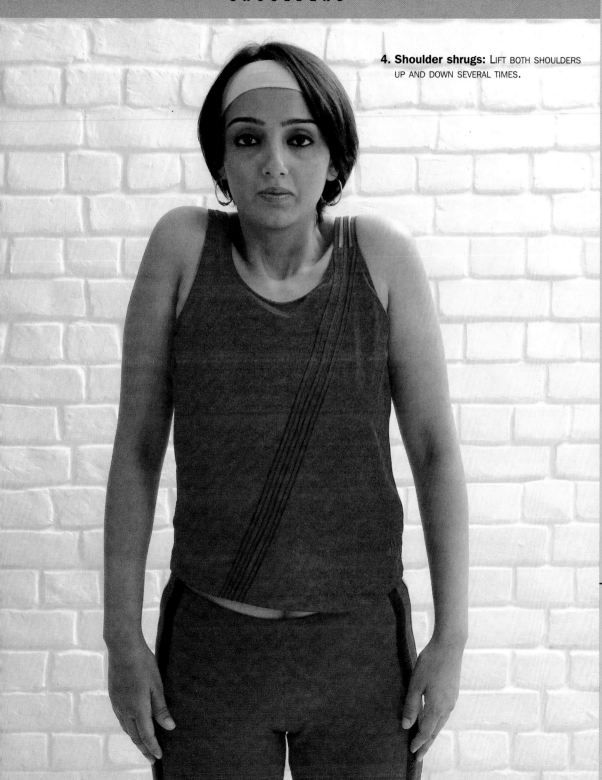

4. Shoulder shrugs: LIFT BOTH SHOULDERS UP AND DOWN SEVERAL TIMES.

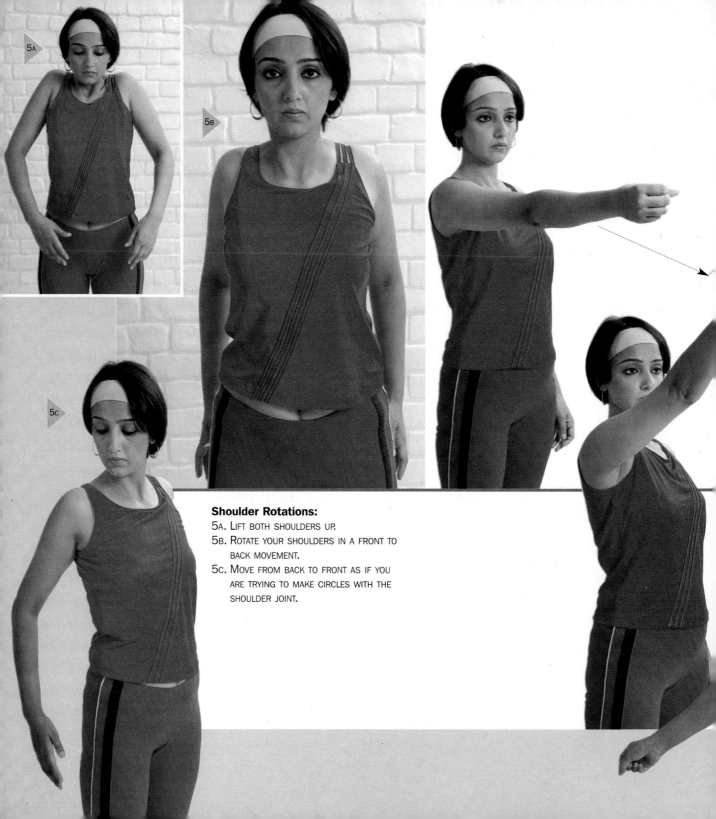

Shoulder Rotations:

5A. LIFT BOTH SHOULDERS UP.

5B. ROTATE YOUR SHOULDERS IN A FRONT TO BACK MOVEMENT.

5C. MOVE FROM BACK TO FRONT AS IF YOU ARE TRYING TO MAKE CIRCLES WITH THE SHOULDER JOINT.

6. Full arm circumduction: DO THIS WITH THE RIGHT ARM FIRST AND THEN WITH THE LEFT. LIGHTLY CLOSE THE FIST AND ROTATE THE ARM IN A FULL CIRCLE FROM FRONT TO BACK AT LEAST EIGHT TIMES AND THEN REVERSE THE MOVEMENT AND REPEAT EIGHT TIMES.

7. Vertical raise: TAKE BOTH ARMS UP AND DOWN SO THAT THE ARMS ALMOST TOUCH YOUR EARS. DO THIS EXERCISE FAST AND AT LEAST 24 TIMES.

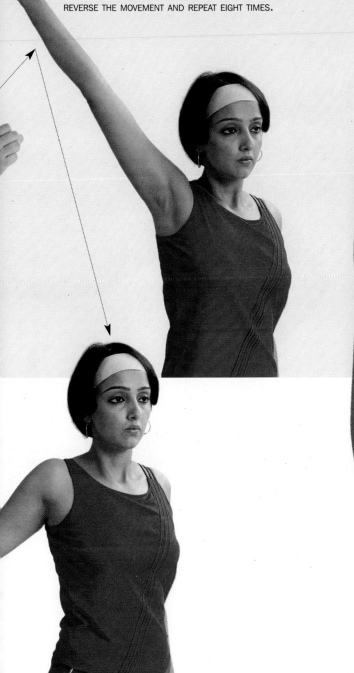

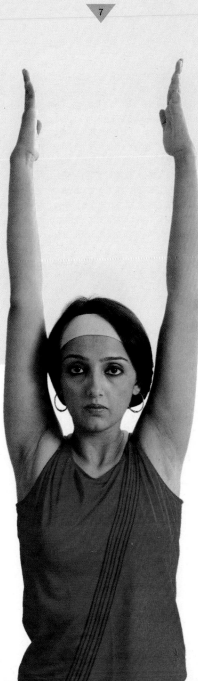

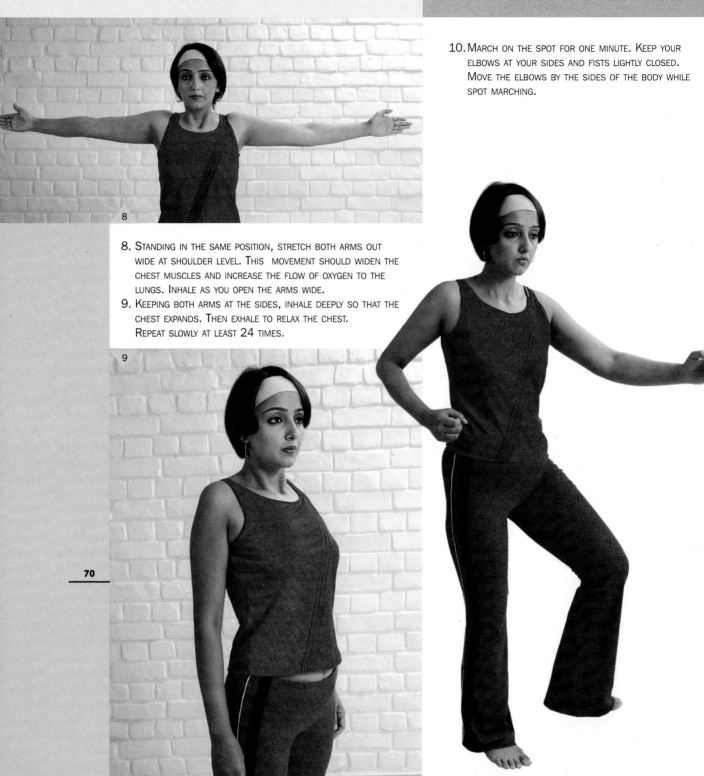

8

8. STANDING IN THE SAME POSITION, STRETCH BOTH ARMS OUT WIDE AT SHOULDER LEVEL. THIS MOVEMENT SHOULD WIDEN THE CHEST MUSCLES AND INCREASE THE FLOW OF OXYGEN TO THE LUNGS. INHALE AS YOU OPEN THE ARMS WIDE.
9. KEEPING BOTH ARMS AT THE SIDES, INHALE DEEPLY SO THAT THE CHEST EXPANDS. THEN EXHALE TO RELAX THE CHEST. REPEAT SLOWLY AT LEAST 24 TIMES.

9

10. MARCH ON THE SPOT FOR ONE MINUTE. KEEP YOUR ELBOWS AT YOUR SIDES AND FISTS LIGHTLY CLOSED. MOVE THE ELBOWS BY THE SIDES OF THE BODY WHILE SPOT MARCHING.

70

11. ADD ON TEN JUMPING JACKS AFTER EVERY TEN MARCHES AND DO THIS INTERVAL CARDIO TRAINING FOR ONE MINUTE.

13. WITH FEET TOGETHER IMITATE TRAMPOLINE JUMPS. DO THIS FOR ONE MINUTE.

WORD OF CAUTION. ALWAYS LAND ON THE BALL OF THE FOOT AND TOUCH THE FULL FOOT TO THE FLOOR BEFORE THE NEXT JUMP OR JOG. ALL POWER MOVES SHOULD BE DONE ON A MAT.

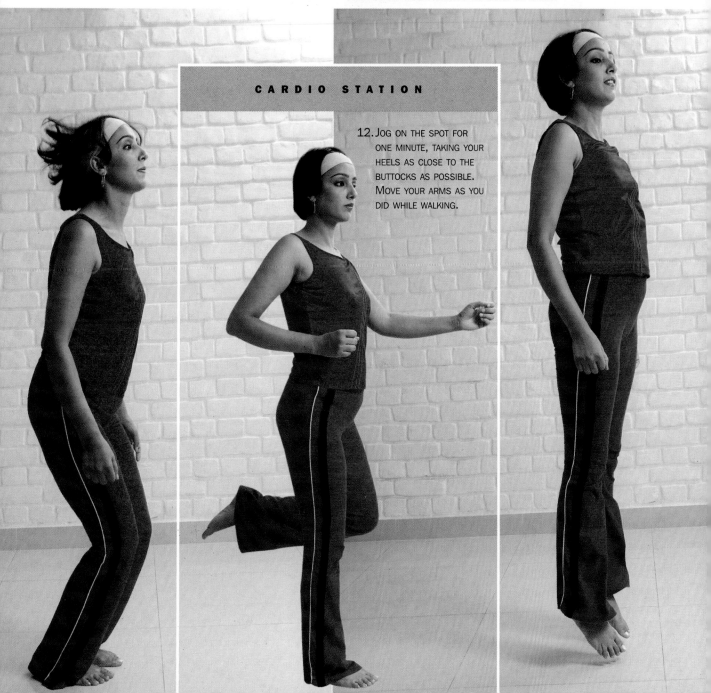

12. JOG ON THE SPOT FOR ONE MINUTE, TAKING YOUR HEELS AS CLOSE TO THE BUTTOCKS AS POSSIBLE. MOVE YOUR ARMS AS YOU DID WHILE WALKING.

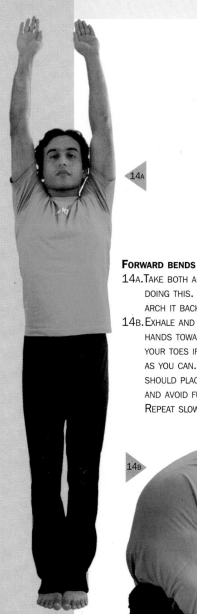

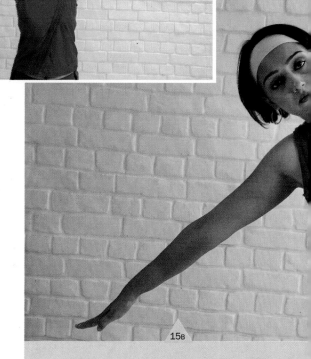

FORWARD BENDS

14A. Take both arms overhead and inhale while doing this. Hyperextend the spine and arch it backwards in this move.

14B. Exhale and bend forward, taking your hands towards the floor. Try and touch your toes if possible, else, only bend as far as you can. (People with back problems should place their hands on their thighs and avoid full forward-bending.) Repeat slowly at least eight times.

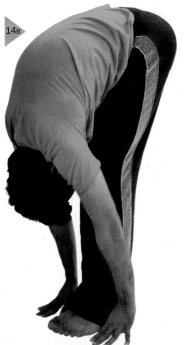

LATERAL BENDS

2A. Extend both arms at shoulder level.

2B. With an exhalation bend the torso to the right. In this position the right palm should point towards the right foot and the left towards the ceiling. Inhale as you return to the starting position.

2C. Repeat on the other side. Hold the lateral bend for a few seconds each time. Repeat 12 times.

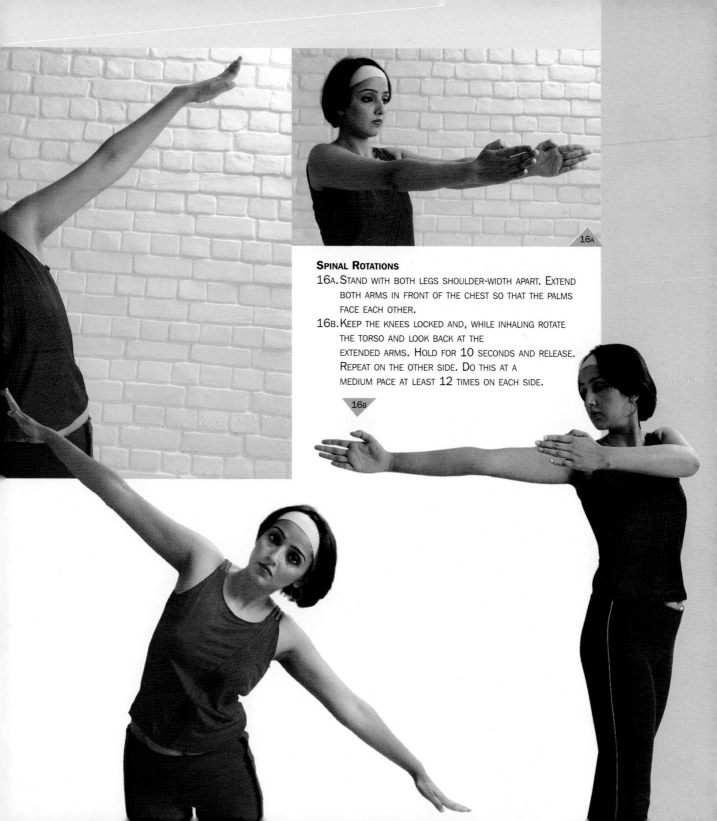

SPINAL ROTATIONS

16A. STAND WITH BOTH LEGS SHOULDER-WIDTH APART. EXTEND BOTH ARMS IN FRONT OF THE CHEST SO THAT THE PALMS FACE EACH OTHER.

16B. KEEP THE KNEES LOCKED AND, WHILE INHALING ROTATE THE TORSO AND LOOK BACK AT THE EXTENDED ARMS. HOLD FOR 10 SECONDS AND RELEASE. REPEAT ON THE OTHER SIDE. DO THIS AT A MEDIUM PACE AT LEAST 12 TIMES ON EACH SIDE.

16A

16B

LEGS

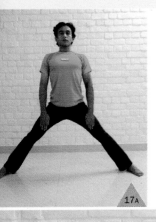

17A. STRETCH THE LEGS AS WIDE AS POSSIBLE, KEEPING YOUR HANDS ON YOUR THIGHS.

17B. EXHALE AND BEND FORWARD, TRYING TO TOUCH BOTH HANDS ON THE FLOOR.

17C. IF THIS LEVEL COMES EASY, THEN PLACE BOTH ELBOWS ON THE FLOOR AND TAKE THE CROWN OF THE HEAD TOWARDS THE FLOOR.

17D. IN THE FINAL STAGE PLACE THE CROWN OF THE HEAD ON THE FLOOR AND HOLD THE ANKLES WITH YOUR HANDS.
FEEL THE STRETCH IN THE HIP JOINT AND THE INNER THIGHS.

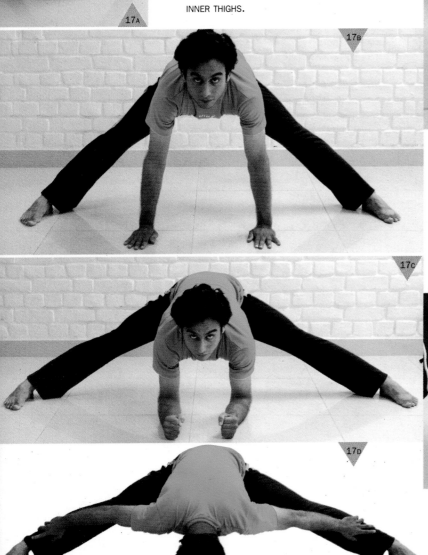

FEET AND ANKLES

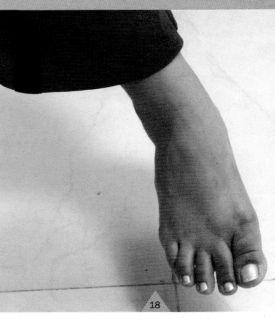

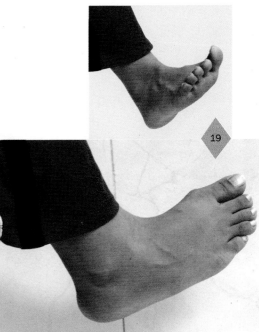

18. POINT AND FLEX THE FEET ONE AT A TIME.
19. ROTATE THE ANKLES CLOCKWISE AND ANTICLOCKWISE. REPEAT EACH EXERCISE 16 TIMES.

STANDING POSTURES

Beginners can practise only the standing postures for at least five weeks.

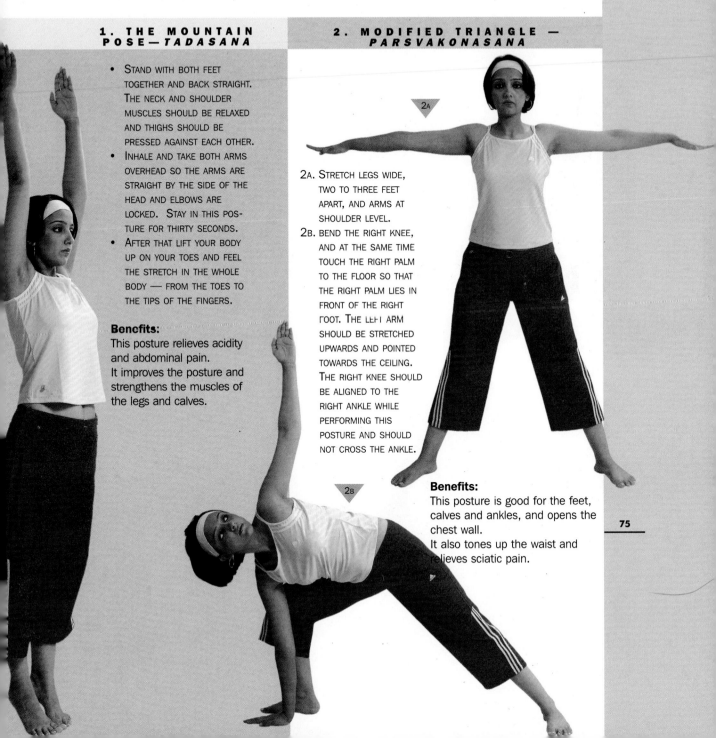

1. THE MOUNTAIN POSE—*TADASANA*

- STAND WITH BOTH FEET TOGETHER AND BACK STRAIGHT. THE NECK AND SHOULDER MUSCLES SHOULD BE RELAXED AND THIGHS SHOULD BE PRESSED AGAINST EACH OTHER.
- INHALE AND TAKE BOTH ARMS OVERHEAD SO THE ARMS ARE STRAIGHT BY THE SIDE OF THE HEAD AND ELBOWS ARE LOCKED. STAY IN THIS POSTURE FOR THIRTY SECONDS.
- AFTER THAT LIFT YOUR BODY UP ON YOUR TOES AND FEEL THE STRETCH IN THE WHOLE BODY — FROM THE TOES TO THE TIPS OF THE FINGERS.

Benefits:
This posture relieves acidity and abdominal pain.
It improves the posture and strengthens the muscles of the legs and calves.

2. MODIFIED TRIANGLE — *PARSVAKONASANA*

2A. STRETCH LEGS WIDE, TWO TO THREE FEET APART, AND ARMS AT SHOULDER LEVEL.

2B. BEND THE RIGHT KNEE, AND AT THE SAME TIME TOUCH THE RIGHT PALM TO THE FLOOR SO THAT THE RIGHT PALM LIES IN FRONT OF THE RIGHT FOOT. THE LEFT ARM SHOULD BE STRETCHED UPWARDS AND POINTED TOWARDS THE CEILING. THE RIGHT KNEE SHOULD BE ALIGNED TO THE RIGHT ANKLE WHILE PERFORMING THIS POSTURE AND SHOULD NOT CROSS THE ANKLE.

Benefits:
This posture is good for the feet, calves and ankles, and opens the chest wall.
It also tones up the waist and relieves sciatic pain.

3. THE TRIANGLE — TRIKONASANA

- KEEP YOUR LEGS TWO TO THREE FEET APART, AND KNEES LOCKED. STRETCH YOUR ARMS OUT AT SHOULDER LEVEL.
- BEND TOWARDS THE RIGHT, TAKING THE RIGHT HAND TOWARDS THE FLOOR AND POINTING THE LEFT ARM TOWARDS THE CEILING. LOOK IN THE DIRECTION OF THE LEFT ARM.

Benefits: This posture is good for toning the legs and removing any minor deformities of the legs. It also relieves backache.

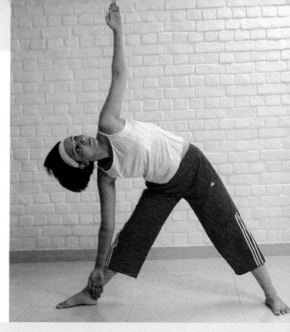

4. THE WARRIOR POSE — VEER ASANA

4A. STARTING WITH BOTH FEET TOGETHER, BACK UPRIGHT AND ARMS PRESSED TO THE SIDES OF THE BODY, TAKE THE RIGHT FOOT FORWARD AND KNEEL ON THE LEFT LEG. CLOSE BOTH FISTS LIGHTLY AND EXTEND THE RIGHT ARM FORWARD.

4B. WITH AN INHALATION, LIFT THE BACK KNEE OFF THE FLOOR, GOING INTO A LUNGE POSITION. THE RIGHT KNEE (THE FORWARD KNEE) SHOULD REMAIN ALIGNED TO THE ANKLE. THE RIGHT ARM SHOULD BE STRETCHED FORWARD AND UP AND THE LEFT HELD TO THE SIDE OF THE BODY. THE EYES SHOULD FOLLOW THE LINE OF THE EXTENDED ARM.

Benefits: This *asana* strengthens the legs and expands the chest. It helps in controlling respiratory ailments and tones up the back.

5. TOE-TOUCHING — PADAHASTA ASANA

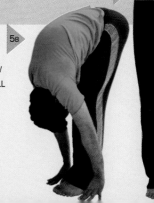

5A. STAND WITH BOTH FEET TOGETHER AND TAKE BOTH ARMS OVERHEAD TO STRETCH BOTH ARMS UPWARDS. INHALE AS YOU TAKE THE ARMS OVERHEAD.

5B. EXHALE AND BEND FORWARD, TAKING THE PALMS DOWN TOWARDS THE FLOOR. GO ONLY AS LOW AS YOU CAN. GRADUALLY THE FLEXIBILITY WILL INCREASE TILL YOU ARE ABLE TO ACHIEVE THE FULL FORWARD BEND AND WILL BE ABLE TO TOUCH YOUR HEAD TO THE KNEES AND PLACE THE PALMS ON THE FLOOR.

FULL FORWARD BENDING SHOULD BE AVOIDED BY PEOPLE WITH BACK PROBLEMS.

Benefits: Toe-touching reduces abdominal fat and lengthens the hamstring muscles. It improves flexibility of the spine.

(SEE PAGE 74, LEGS)

- STAND WITH BOTH LEGS STRETCHED WIDE APART AND FEET POINTED FORWARD.
- WITH AN EXHALATION PLACE BOTH PALMS ON THE FLOOR.
- SLOWLY INCREASE THE STRETCH TO PLACE BOTH ELBOWS ON THE FLOOR.
- FINALLY PLACE THE CROWN OF THE HEAD ON THE FLOOR.
- IF COMFORTABLE, TRY AND HOLD THE ANKLES AND SUPPORT THE BODY ON THE CROWN OF HE HEAD AND THE FEET. BOTH KNEES SHOULD BE TIGHT AND THE BACK STRETCHED. KEEP THE EYES OPEN AND BREATHING NORMAL.

Benefits: This posture stretches the inner thighs and the hamstring muscles at the back of the thighs. It improves digestion and increases the supply of oxygen to the brain.

BALANCING POSTURES

BALANCE IS AN ESSENTIAL PART OF ANY YOGA PROGRAM AND THE FOLLOWING POSTURES WILL HELP TO IMPROVE YOUR BALANCE. YOU CAN TAKE THE SUPPORT OF THE WALL IN THE BEGINNING, BUT LEAVE THIS EXTERNAL SUPPORT AS YOUR BALANCE IMPROVES. IT IS IMPORTANT TO REMEMBER THAT THIS ASPECT OF FITNESS TAKES TIME TO DEVELOP AND GENERALLY DIFFERS FROM THE RIGHT TO THE LEFT SIDE. **EXECUTE EACH POSTURE ONCE ON EACH SIDE.**

1. THE TREE— *VRUKSHASANA*

- STAND WITH BOTH FEET TOGETHER AND ARMS PRESSED TO THE SIDE. THE CHIN SHOULD BE PARALLEL TO THE FLOOR, THE ABDOMEN TIGHT AND INNER THIGHS PRESSED TOGETHER.
- FOLD THE LEFT LEG TO PLACE THE LEFT FOOT AGAINST THE RIGHT INNER THIGH. THE FOOT SHOULD BE HIGH UP ON THE INNER THIGH AND THE FOLDED KNEE SHOULD POINT OUTWARDS. TAKE BOTH ARMS OVERHEAD AND JOIN THE PALMS TOGETHER. MAKE SURE THE ELBOWS ARE LOCKED AND THE ARMS ARE STRAIGHT. FOCUS ON ANY ONE POINT TO MAINTAIN THE POSTURE FOR AT LEAST A MINUTE. REPEAT WITH THE OTHER LEG.

Benefits: This posture tones the muscles of the legs and improves both poise and posture.

2. THE KITE POSE — *PATANGASANA*

- STAND WITH FEET TOGETHER AND TAKE THE LEFT LEG BACK AND UP. EXHALE AND BEND FORWARD FROM THE HIP JOINT. THE BODY SHOULD BE IN A STRAIGHT LINE.
- STRETCH BOTH ARMS TO SHOULDER LEVEL AND KEEP THE NECK IN LINE WITH THE REST OF THE SPINE. TUCK THE ABDOMEN IN. HOLD FROM 10 TO 60 SECONDS. REPEAT WITH THE OTHER LEG. MAINTAIN NORMAL BREATHING.

Benefits: This posture improves balance and strengthens the legs, back and abdomen.

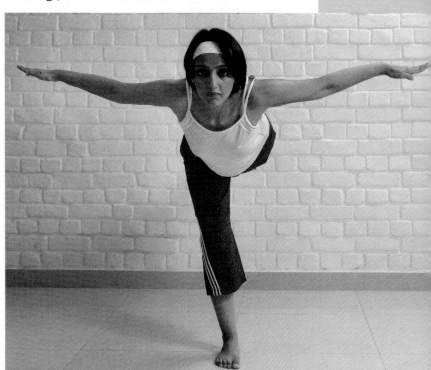

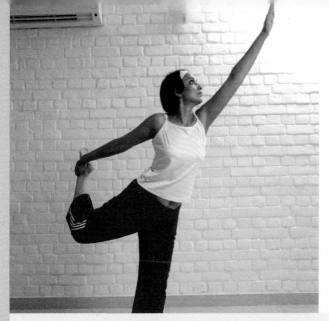

3. THE DANCING LORD POSTURE — ARDHANATRAJASANA

- STAND WITH BOTH FEET TOGETHER AND FLEX THE RIGHT KNEE S THAT THE RIGHT HEEL IS RAISED NEAR THE RIGHT BUTTOCK.
- EXTEND THE LEFT ARM IN FRONT AND WITH THE RIGHT HAND, HOLD THE ANKLE OF THE FOLDED LEG AND STRETCH IT BACK AN UP. KEEP THE LEFT KNEE STRAIGHT AND BACK TALL. HOLD FOR 10 TO 60 SECONDS.
- REPEAT WITH THE OTHER LEG.

Benefits: This posture stretches the hip flexor muscles improves balance and strengthens the legs.

SITTING POSTURES

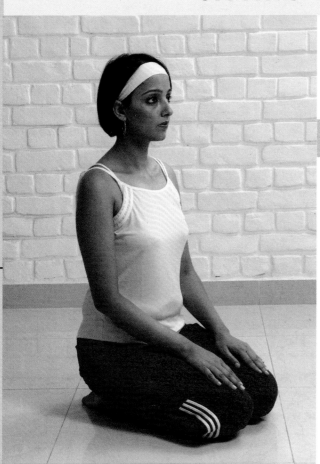

Sit with both legs stretched forward and keep the back tall. To change from one exercise to another revert to this starting position. Repeat once on each side.

1. SITTING ON THE HEELS — VAJRASANA

SIT ON FOLDED KNEES AND FLATTEN THE HEELS SO THAT THE BUTTOCKS ARE RESTING ON THE HEELS. IN THE BEGINNING THIS MAY SEEM A BIT TOUGH AS THE MUSCLES AT THE TOP OF THE FEET AND THE ANKLE JOINTS ARE STIFF, BUT GRADUALLY THE STIFFNESS WILL GO AWAY AND SITTING WILL BECOME EASIER. THIS STANCE SHOULD BE HELD FOR AT LEAST ONE MINUTE.
THIS IS THE ONLY ASANA ONE CAN DO IMMEDIATELY AFTER A MEAL.

Benefits: If done regularly, it aids digestion and the general well-being of the digestive system. It also prevents accumulation of fat.

2. THE TORTOISE POSE — *KURMASANA*

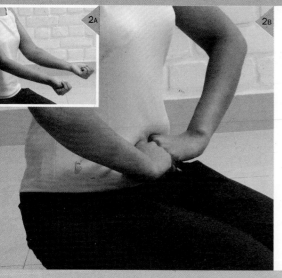

2A. SIT IN THE POSTURE FOR *VAJRASANA*. CLOSE BOTH FISTS BY PLACING THE THUMB INSIDE THE PALM.

2B. PLACE THE CLOSED FIST ON EITHER SIDE OF THE NAVEL BUT DO NOT BLOCK THE NAVEL. PUT GENTLE PRESSURE ON THE INTESTINAL WALL AND INHALE DEEPLY TO EXPAND YOUR STOMACH.

2C. BEND FORWARD WITH AN EXHALATION AND LOOK FORWARD. KEEP THE HIPS IN CONTACT WITH THE HEEL IF POSSIBLE. THIS POSTURE WILL IMPROVE WITH PRACTICE. HOLD FOR A FEW SECONDS AND RELEASE WITH AN INHALATION.

Benefits: This posture aids digestion, prevents gas formation and other stress-related digestive disorders.

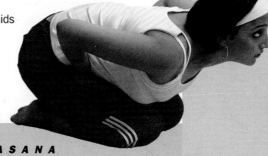

3. THE CAMEL POSE — *USHTRASANA*

3A. SIT IN A KNEELING POSITION AND KEEP THE FEET FLAT ON THE FLOOR OR ON THE TOES. THIS WILL DEPEND ON THE FLEXIBILITY OF YOUR BODY AND YOUR ABILITY TO DO THE CAMEL POSTURE. KEEP THE LEGS APART IN THE BEGINNING.

3B. FOR A COMPLETE BEGINNER IT IS IMPORTANT TO PROGRESS SLOWLY BY INHALING AND BENDING BACK TO PLACE THE RIGHT HAND ON THE RIGHT HEEL; THE LEFT ARM SHOULD BE HELD STRAIGHT UP. REPEAT ON THE OTHER SIDE.

3C. AS THE FLEXIBILITY OF THE SPINE IMPROVES, TAKE BOTH HANDS SIMULTANEOUSLY BEHIND AND BEND BACK FROM THE NECK TO THE NAVEL. KEEP THE BREATHING NORMAL WHILE HOLDING THE POSTURE AND THE EYES OPEN. HOLD THE POSTURE FOR 10 TO 60 SECONDS. EXHALE AS YOU RELEASE THE POSTURE.

Benefits: This pose stretches the abdominal wall, opens the chest (thoracic cavity), is good for respiratory ailments and strengthens the muscles of the back.

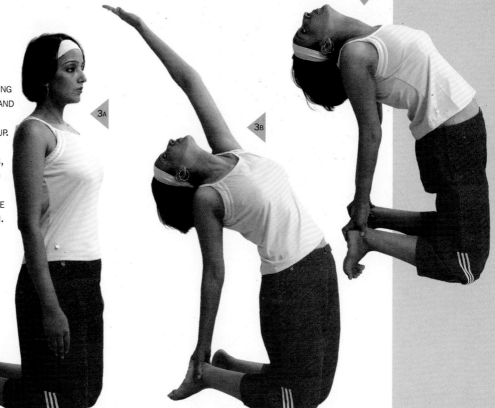

4. HEAD TO KNEE STRETCH— JANUSHIRSHASAN

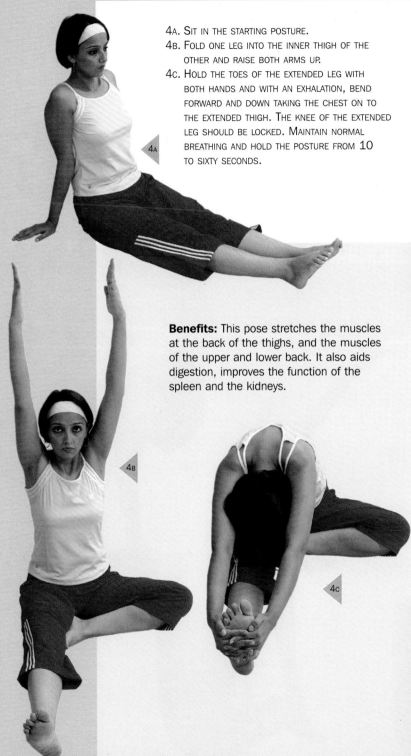

4A. SIT IN THE STARTING POSTURE.

4B. FOLD ONE LEG INTO THE INNER THIGH OF THE OTHER AND RAISE BOTH ARMS UP.

4C. HOLD THE TOES OF THE EXTENDED LEG WITH BOTH HANDS AND WITH AN EXHALATION, BEND FORWARD AND DOWN TAKING THE CHEST ON TO THE EXTENDED THIGH. THE KNEE OF THE EXTENDED LEG SHOULD BE LOCKED. MAINTAIN NORMAL BREATHING AND HOLD THE POSTURE FROM 10 TO SIXTY SECONDS.

Benefits: This pose stretches the muscles at the back of the thighs, and the muscles of the upper and lower back. It also aids digestion, improves the function of the spleen and the kidneys.

5. THE BUTTERFLY — BHADRASANA

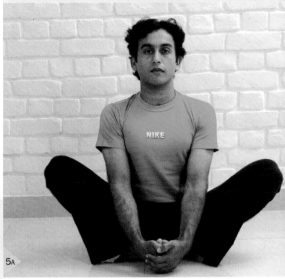

5A. SIT IN THE STARTING POSITION WITH BOTH LEGS STRETCHED FORWARD AND STRAIGHT.

• FOLD BOTH KNEES AND PLACE THE SOLE OF ONE FOOT AGAINST THE OTHER AND SPREAD BOTH KNEES WIDE AND DOWN TOWARDS THE FLOOR.

• FLAP THE KNEES UP AND DOWN QUICKLY LIKE THE WINGS OF A BUTTERFLY. IN THE BEGINNING THIS MAY BE DIFFICULT IF THE LIGAMENTS IN THE HIP JOINT ARE TIGHT BUT THE RANGE OF MOTION WILL IMPROVE WITH PRACTICE. TO BEGIN WITH, JUST KEEP THE BACK TALL AND KNEES DOWN.

5B. AFTER A FEW WEEKS, TRY AND BEND FORWARD TO TAKE THE CHEST TOWARDS THE FLOOR.

Benefits: This is a very good *asana* for the organs and muscles of the pelvic floor. It maintains the health of the reproductive system and eases menstrual cramps in women.

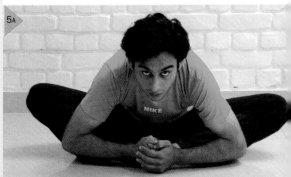

- Stretch both legs wide and try and hold the toes with the hands.
- Exhale and slowly bend forward and down, taking the chest towards the floor.

In the beginning just stretch the legs wide and keep the back tall. The rest can follow slowly. Hold from ten to sixty seconds.

Benefits: This is good for the reproductive organs and helps to improve the flexibility of the hip joint.

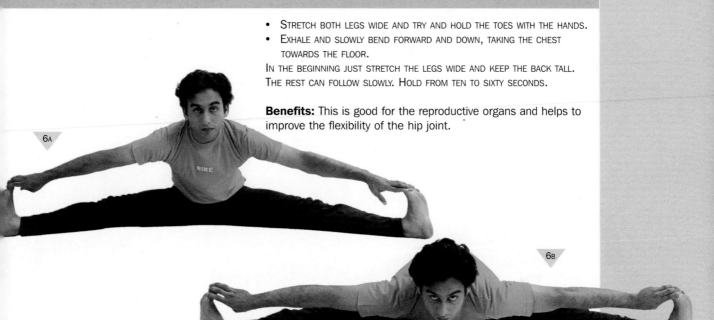

7. BACK STRETCH — *PASCHIMUTTANASANA*

7A. Sit with both legs extended forward and hold the toes of the extended feet.

7B. Exhale, pull in the abdomen and bend forward and down, taking the chest towards the thighs. You may not be able to go very low in the beginning but the flexibility will improve with regular practice. Inhale as you release the posture. (People with back problems should not bend forward.)

Benefits: This improves the function of the digestive and the renal systems and tones the abdominal wall.

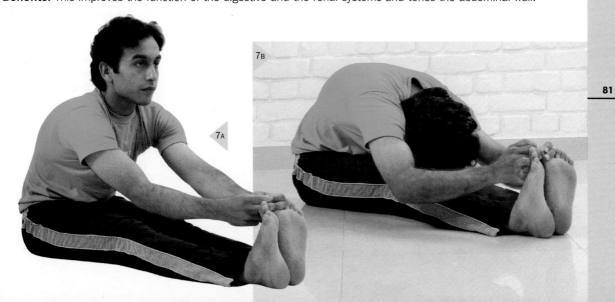

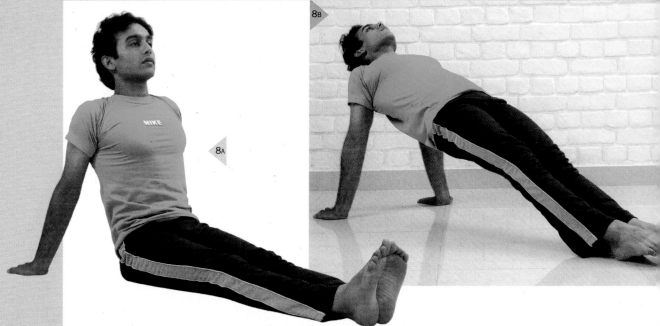

8A. SIT WITH BOTH LEGS EXTENDED FORWARD.
* PLACE BOTH ARMS BEHIND THE HIPS AND KEEP THEM SHOULDER-WIDTH APART. KEEP THE PALMS SLIGHTLY OPEN AND FINGERS POINTING BACK. THE SHOULDER BLADES SHOULD BE RETRACTED OR PULLED TOWARDS EACH OTHER AND THE ABDOMEN AND HIPS HELD TIGHT.

8B. WITH AN INHALATION LIFT THE WHOLE BODY UP IN A SLANT AND LET THE NECK STAY BACK, YET ALIGNED TO THE SPINE. THE WEIGHT OF THE BODY SHOULD REST ON THE ARMS. THERE SHOULD NOT BE ANY COMPRESSION OF THE WRIST. IF POSSIBLE TRY AND TOUCH THE TOES TO THE FLOOR, EXTENDING THE FEET COMPLETELY.

Benefits: THIS POSTURE RELIEVES THE STRESS CAUSED BY FORWARD BENDING POSTURES. IT STRENGTHENS THE SHOULDERS, WRISTS AND THE ANKLES, AND EXPANDS THE LUNGS AND THE CHEST. **THIS CAN AND SHOULD BE DONE BY PEOPLE WITH BACK PROBLEMS.**

NOTE

Yoga is all about balancing the opposites. A forward-bending posture will have a complimentary back-bending one
This is to balance the shifting of the spinal fluid (in the spinal discs) from the front to the back and vice versa
to maintain the health and strength of the discs. This rule is applicable to the lateral bends as well.

Breathing usually follows a simple rule. Any forward bending or lateral bending requires exhalation
and any hyperextension of the back or back-bending requires inhalation.

Holding a posture from 10 to 60 seconds is advised
to help improve the flexibility of joints and the length of the muscles.

9. SEATED SPINAL TWIST — *ARDHAMACHENDRA ASANA*

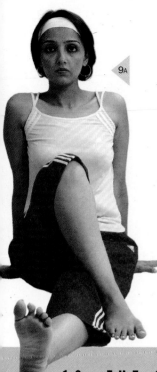

Named after a holy man, this is a posture with spinal rotation to maintain the flexibility of the vertebrae and to exercise the small muscles of the spine. These muscles — the multifidus — are small and strong, and hold the vertebrae together.

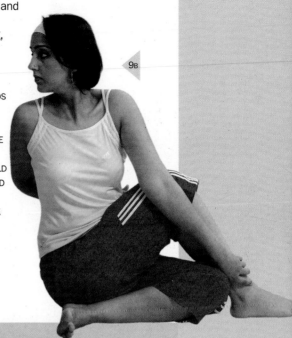

9A. SIT WITH BOTH LEGS EXTENDED FORWARD.
- FOLD THE RIGHT LEG SO THAT THE KNEE POINTS TOWARDS THE CEILING.
- CROSS THIS LEG OVER THE LEFT THIGH.

9B. FOLD THE LEFT LEG SO THAT THE LEFT HEEL STAYS CLOSE TO THE RIGHT HIP.
- EXTEND THE LEFT ARM ACROSS THE RIGHT THIGH TO HOLD THE RIGHT FOOT OR ANKLE, WHILE THE LEFT ARM SHOULD BE CURLED AROUND THE SPINE. LOOK OVER THE RIGHT SHOULDER TO MAKE A SPINAL ROTATION FROM THE NECK TO THE LOWER BACK.

Benefits: This posture is beneficial in controlling diabetes and improves the digestive system as well. It also exercises the spine.

10. THE COW FACE POSE — *GOMUKHASANA*

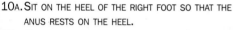

10A. SIT ON THE HEEL OF THE RIGHT FOOT SO THAT THE ANUS RESTS ON THE HEEL.

10B. CROSS THE LEFT LEG OVER THE RIGHT THIGH TO REST THE LEFT KNEE ON THE RIGHT AND THE LEFT FOOT TO REST ALONGSIDE THE RIGHT HIP.

10C. TAKE THE LEFT ARM UP AND BEHIND SO THE LEFT PALM RESTS BETWEEN THE SHOULDER BLADES.
- TWIST THE RIGHT ARM AND TAKE IT BEHIND THE BACK TO HOLD THE LEFT PALM. THE NECK SHOULD BE STRAIGHT AND THERE SHOULD BE NO TENSION AROUND THE NECK AND SHOULDER AREA.
  REPEAT ON THE OTHER SIDE.

Note. If the seating posture is difficult to achieve then this exercise can be done by sitting in *VAJRASANA* or simply by sitting on flattened heels. The flexibility of the shoulder joint may be less on any one side. This is quite normal and will improve with practice.

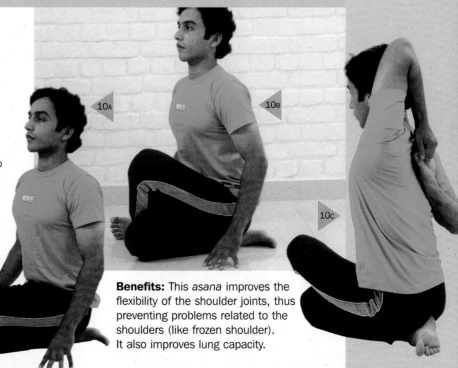

Benefits: This *asana* improves the flexibility of the shoulder joints, thus preventing problems related to the shoulders (like frozen shoulder). It also improves lung capacity.

11. THE RABBIT POSE — SHASHANKASANA

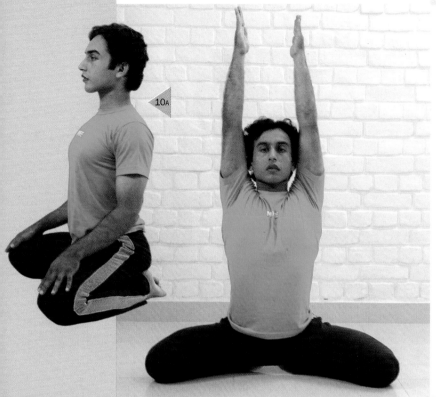

10A

11A. Sit on flattened feet and open both knees as wide as possible.
11B. Take both arms overhead with an inhalation.
11C. Exhale and bend forward, taking the chest towards the floor. This is one forward bending posture that can be done by all — even people with back problems.

Benefits: This stretches the spine, removing any stress on it.

84

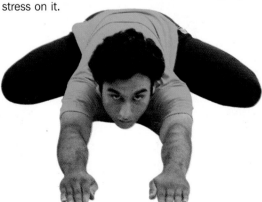

12. THE LION POSE — SIMHASANA

12A. Maintain the same posture as the rabbit but lift the torso up and rest the palms in front of the knees.
• Hollow the lumbar spine and turn the neck and face upwards to look at the ceiling.
12B. Open the mouth wide and extend the tongue out fully, exhaling loudly (imitating the roar of a lion). Repeat at least 12 times. With every exhalation feel the contraction in the abdominal muscles and pull the navel towards the spine.

Benefits: This posture is an excellent stress buster. It also tones the vocal cords and exercises the throat.

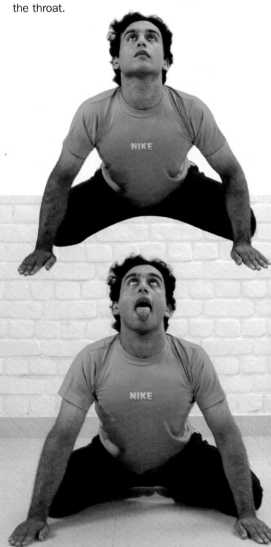

ACUTE OR CHRONIC BACKACHE CAN BE DUE TO SEVERAL REASONS OTHER THAN INJURY OR AGE-RELATED WEAR AND TEAR OF THE VERTEBRAE. STRESS, BAD POSTURE, USE OF AN UNCOMFORTABLE MATTRESS OR CHAIR, EXCESS WEIGHT AROUND THE MIDDLE, BAD LIFTING/CARRYING TECHNIQUES, AND GENETIC DEFORMITIES CAN BE THE CAUSE OF A BACKACHE.

YOGA POSTURES DEAL WITH THE CONDITION IN A WHOLESOME MANNER BY SUGGESTING EXERCISES TO TONE AND STRENGTHEN THE ABDOMEN AND BACK AND A WHOLESOME DIET TO TAKE OFF THE EXTRA POUNDS. ADDING MEDITATION TO THE EXERCISE PROGRAMME WILL RELIEVE STRESS AND REMOVE THE ROOT CAUSE OF EATING DISORDERS AND UNEXPLAINED BACKACHE.

Supine postures should be done with caution and only after the initial standing and sitting postures have been practised for five to six weeks.

SUPINE POSTURES

THE STARTING POSITION FOR SUPINE POSTURES IS TO LIE, FACE UP. ARMS SHOULD BE BY THE SIDE OF THE HIPS WITH PALMS PRESSED TO THE FLOOR. THE NECK MUST BE NATURALLY ALIGNED WITH A SLIGHT ARCH IN BETWEEN THE NECK AND SHOULDER AREA AND THE NATURAL LUMBAR CURVE (OF THE LOWER BACK TO BE MAINTAINED AT ALL TIMES). FOCUSED BREATHING IS NECESSARY AT ALL TIMES. HOLD EACH POSTURE FROM 10 TO 60 SECONDS OR MORE, WITHOUT COMPROMISING THE BODY ALIGNMENT.

ALL SUPINE POSTURES STRENGTHEN THE ABDOMINAL WALL AND KEEP THE WAIST TRIM. INTERNALLY ALL THESE POSTURES AID AND IMPROVE DIGESTION AND RELIEVE PROBLEMS RELATED TO DIGESTION.

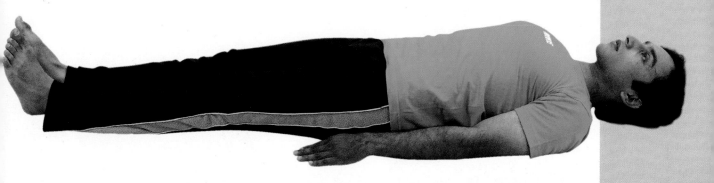

1. STRAIGHT LEG LIFT — *UTTANPADASANA*

1A. BEGINNERS SHOULD LIFT ONE LEG AT A TIME. PEOPLE WITH STRONGER ABDOMINAL MUSCLES CAN LIFT BOTH LEGS OFF THE FLOOR SIMULTANEOUSLY WHILE INHALING. THE LEG LIFT SHOULD INVOLVE THE USE OF ABDOMINAL MUSCLES MORE THAN THE HIP FLEXORS OR THE OTHER MUSCLES OF THE LEG.

1B. TRY AND KEEP THE LEGS STRAIGHT UP WITH FEET POINTING TOWARDS THE CEILING, THE NAVEL PULLED TOWARDS THE SPINE AND KNEES AS STRAIGHT AS POSSIBLE. FEEL THE CONTRACTION IN THE ABDOMINAL WALL LIKE YOU ARE WEARING A TIGHT PAIR OF JEANS. ONCE THE POSTURE IS ATTAINED, MAINTAIN THE NORMAL BREATHING PATTERN AND HOLD THE POSTURE.
IF HOLDING THE POSTURE IS NOT POSSIBLE IN THE BEGINNING THEN REPEAT THE EXERCISE THREE TO FIVE TIMES SLOWLY.

1C. BRING THE LEGS DOWN VERY SLOWLY AND WITHOUT OVERARCHING THE SPINE IN THE CERVICAL OR THE LUMBAR REGION. PROGRESSION TO THE EXERCISE IS TO TAKE BOTH LEGS HALF WAY DOWN AND HOLD THE POSITION WITHOUT THE SPINE OVERARCHING.

1D. THE FINAL PROGRESSION WOULD BE TO HOLD THE FEET JUST ABOUT 6 INCHES ABOVE THE FLOOR WHILE MAINTAINING THE SPINAL ALIGNMENT.

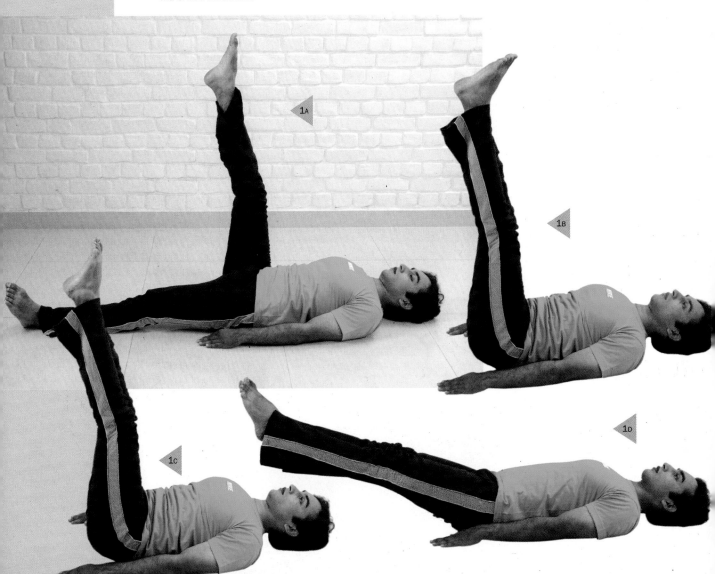

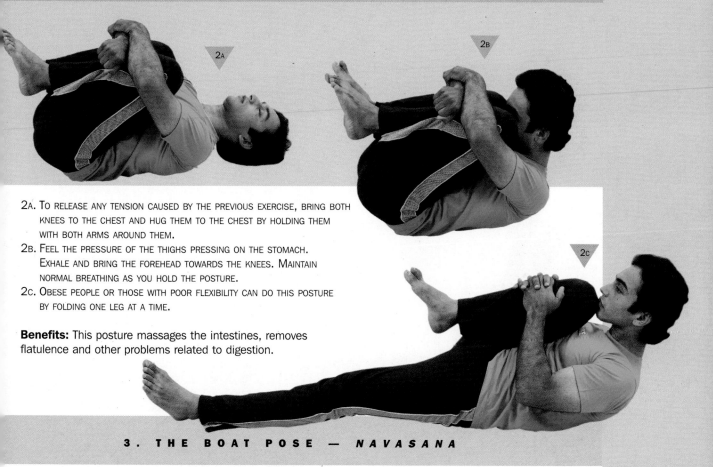

2A. TO RELEASE ANY TENSION CAUSED BY THE PREVIOUS EXERCISE, BRING BOTH
KNEES TO THE CHEST AND HUG THEM TO THE CHEST BY HOLDING THEM
WITH BOTH ARMS AROUND THEM.

2B. FEEL THE PRESSURE OF THE THIGHS PRESSING ON THE STOMACH.
EXHALE AND BRING THE FOREHEAD TOWARDS THE KNEES. MAINTAIN
NORMAL BREATHING AS YOU HOLD THE POSTURE.

2C. OBESE PEOPLE OR THOSE WITH POOR FLEXIBILITY CAN DO THIS POSTURE
BY FOLDING ONE LEG AT A TIME.

Benefits: This posture massages the intestines, removes
flatulence and other problems related to digestion.

3. THE BOAT POSE — *NAVASANA*

AS THE ABDOMINAL WALL BECOMES STRONGER, THIS POSTURE CAN BE ATTEMPTED.
TAKE THE STARTING POSITION ON THE MAT AND WHILE INHALING, LIFT THE HEAD, NECK, SHOULDERS AND LEGS AND ARMS ABOUT ONE
FOOT FROM THE FLOOR SIMULTANEOUSLY AND BALANCE THE BODY ON THE LOWER BACK. IN THIS THE SACRUM (LOWER BACK) SHOULD
BE IN CONTACT WITH THE FLOOR AND THE ABDOMEN SHOULD BE HELD IN AND TIGHTENED. SHOULDER BLADES SHOULD BE DOWN AND
BACK AND THERE SHOULD BE NO TENSION AROUND THE NECK AND SHOULDERS. THE SHOULDER SHOULD NOT HUNCH UP AND THE
NORMAL DISTANCE BETWEEN THE EARS AND THE SHOULDERS SHOULD BE MAINTAINED AT ALL TIMES. BOTH ARMS SHOULD BE STRAIGHT
AND JUST ABOVE THE THIGHS.

RELEASE THE POSTURE AND RELAX IN
SAVASANA (SEE PAGE 59) TO GET RID
OF ANY STRESS CAUSED DURING
THE EXECUTION OF THIS POSTURE.

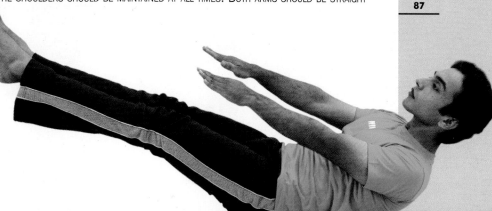

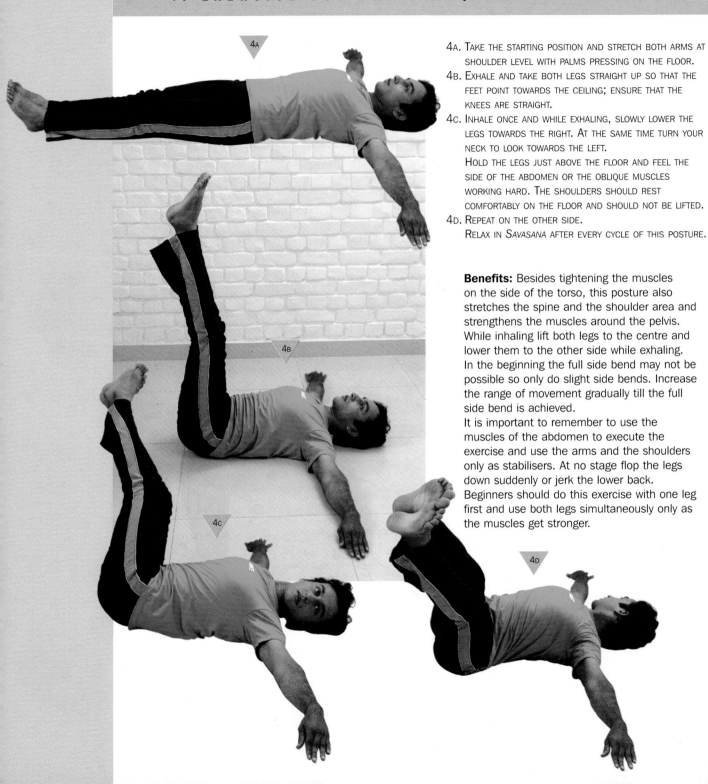

4A. TAKE THE STARTING POSITION AND STRETCH BOTH ARMS AT SHOULDER LEVEL WITH PALMS PRESSING ON THE FLOOR.

4B. EXHALE AND TAKE BOTH LEGS STRAIGHT UP SO THAT THE FEET POINT TOWARDS THE CEILING; ENSURE THAT THE KNEES ARE STRAIGHT.

4C. INHALE ONCE AND WHILE EXHALING, SLOWLY LOWER THE LEGS TOWARDS THE RIGHT. AT THE SAME TIME TURN YOUR NECK TO LOOK TOWARDS THE LEFT.
HOLD THE LEGS JUST ABOVE THE FLOOR AND FEEL THE SIDE OF THE ABDOMEN OR THE OBLIQUE MUSCLES WORKING HARD. THE SHOULDERS SHOULD REST COMFORTABLY ON THE FLOOR AND SHOULD NOT BE LIFTED.

4D. REPEAT ON THE OTHER SIDE.
RELAX IN *SAVASANA* AFTER EVERY CYCLE OF THIS POSTURE.

Benefits: Besides tightening the muscles on the side of the torso, this posture also stretches the spine and the shoulder area and strengthens the muscles around the pelvis. While inhaling lift both legs to the centre and lower them to the other side while exhaling. In the beginning the full side bend may not be possible so only do slight side bends. Increase the range of movement gradually till the full side bend is achieved.

It is important to remember to use the muscles of the abdomen to execute the exercise and use the arms and the shoulders only as stabilisers. At no stage flop the legs down suddenly or jerk the lower back. Beginners should do this exercise with one leg first and use both legs simultaneously only as the muscles get stronger.

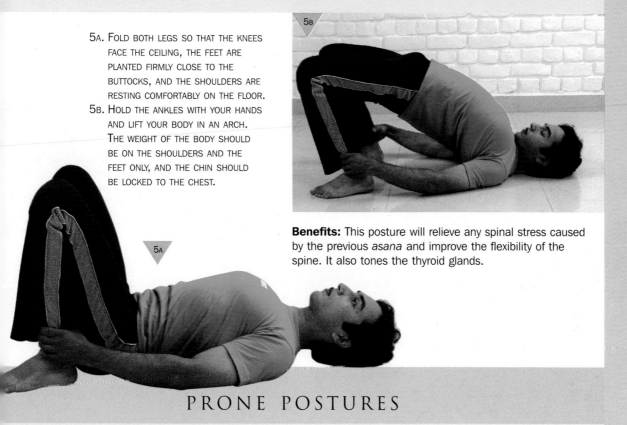

5A. FOLD BOTH LEGS SO THAT THE KNEES FACE THE CEILING, THE FEET ARE PLANTED FIRMLY CLOSE TO THE BUTTOCKS, AND THE SHOULDERS ARE RESTING COMFORTABLY ON THE FLOOR.

5B. HOLD THE ANKLES WITH YOUR HANDS AND LIFT YOUR BODY IN AN ARCH. THE WEIGHT OF THE BODY SHOULD BE ON THE SHOULDERS AND THE FEET ONLY, AND THE CHIN SHOULD BE LOCKED TO THE CHEST.

Benefits: This posture will relieve any spinal stress caused by the previous *asana* and improve the flexibility of the spine. It also tones the thyroid glands.

PRONE POSTURES

FOR PRONE POSTURES THE STARTING POSITION IS FACE DOWN ON THE EXERCISE MAT WITH THE FOREHEAD TOUCHING THE MAT, ARMS BY THE SIDE OF THE BODY, AND PALMS PRESSING ON THE FLOOR.

BENEFITS OF THESE POSTURES ARE FOR STRENGTHENING THE MUSCLES OF THE BACK AND STRETCHING THE ABDOMINAL AND CHEST WALL. THESE POSTURES ALSO IMPROVE THE HEALTH AND STRENGTH OF THE INTERVERTEBRAL DISCS.

EACH POSTURE SHOULD BE HELD FROM 10 TO 60 SECONDS BUT THE PROGRESS SHOULD BE SLOW AND SYSTEMATIC AS WITH ALL THE OTHER POSTURES.

FOR ALL POSTURES IN THE PRONE POSITION, INHALE WHILE TAKING THE POSTURE AND EXHALE WHILE RELEASING THE POSTURE.

NORMALLY WE NEVER DO ANY BACK-BENDING ACTIVITIES/EXERCISES IN OUR DAILY LIFE. MOST OF OUR CHORES INVOLVE ONLY FORWARD BENDING. DOING THESE *ASANAS* WILL MAKE THE SPINE MORE FLEXIBLE AND REMOVE THE PROBLEMS ASSOCIATED WITH STOOPING SHOULDERS (KYPHOSIS) AND ROUNDED BACK, STIFFNESS IN THE BACK DUE TO INACTIVITY, POOR MUSCULAR STRENGTH AND A SLIPPED DISC.

CAUTION. PEOPLE WITH HYPERTENSION SHOULD NOT HOLD THESE POSTURES FOR TOO LONG.

1. EASY POSTURE — *SALABHASANA*

1A. PLACE BOTH PALMS IN LINE WITH THE CHEST, FEET TOGETHER AND FLAT ON THE FLOOR AND FOREHEAD TOUCHING THE FLOOR.

1B. WHILE INHALING, LIFT THE HANDS, HEAD, SHOULDERS AND CHEST FROM THE FLOOR. ALL THE WEIGHT SHOULD REST ON THE ABDOMINAL WALL. THE SHOULDER BLADES SHOULD BE PULLED BACK AND DOWN AND ELBOWS SHOULD BE CLOSE BY THE SIDE OF THE BODY, WITH BOTH PALMS LIFTED FROM THE FLOOR. MAINTAIN NORMAL BREATHING.

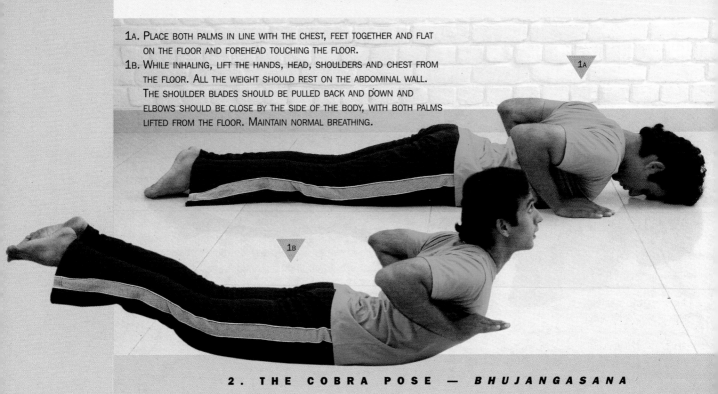

2. THE COBRA POSE — *BHUJANGASANA*

2A. PLACE THE PALMS IN LINE WITH THE CHEST AND TOUCH THE FOREHEAD TO THE FLOOR. BOTH FEET SHOULD BE TOGETHER AND FLAT ON THE FLOOR.

2B. INHALE AND PUSH THE UPPER BODY AWAY FROM THE FLOOR AND STRAIGHTEN THE ELBOWS FULLY, LOOKING UP TOWARDS THE CEILING. IN THE BEGINNING A FULL STRETCH MAY BE DIFFICULT, SO KEEP THE ELBOWS BENT IF REQUIRED.

NOTE. THE FULL *BHUJANGASANA* WILL BE POSSIBLE ONLY WITH REGULAR PRACTICE. IN THE FINAL POSTURE THE SPINE SHOULD BE A FULL CURVE FROM THE NECK TO THE TAILBONE, WITH THE HIP BONE TOUCHING THE FLOOR, THE INNER THIGHS PRESSED TOGETHER AND THE FEET FLAT.

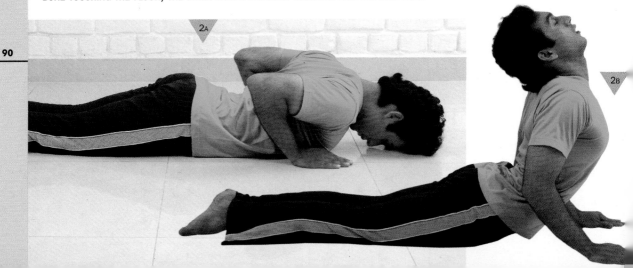

3. THE BOW POSE — *DHANURASANA*

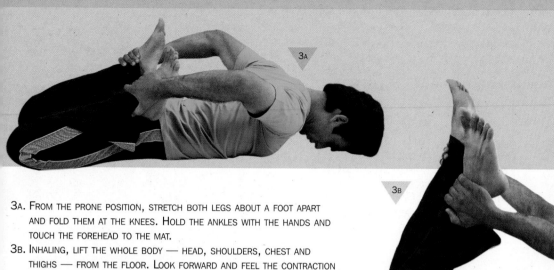

3A. FROM THE PRONE POSITION, STRETCH BOTH LEGS ABOUT A FOOT APART AND FOLD THEM AT THE KNEES. HOLD THE ANKLES WITH THE HANDS AND TOUCH THE FOREHEAD TO THE MAT.

3B. INHALING, LIFT THE WHOLE BODY — HEAD, SHOULDERS, CHEST AND THIGHS — FROM THE FLOOR. LOOK FORWARD AND FEEL THE CONTRACTION IN THE MUSCLES OF THE BACK WHILE ALL THE MUSCLES IN THE FRONT OF THE BODY ARE STRETCHED OUT. LIFT HIGHER AS THE FLEXIBILITY INCREASES AND HOLD FOR A LONGER TIME.

BENEFITS: THIS *ASANA* WILL NOT ONLY STRENGTHEN THE BACK BUT ALSO STRENGTHEN THE ARMS. IT WILL STRETCH ALL THE MUSCLES IN THE FRONT OF THE BODY.

4. BOAT POSE — *NAUKASANA*

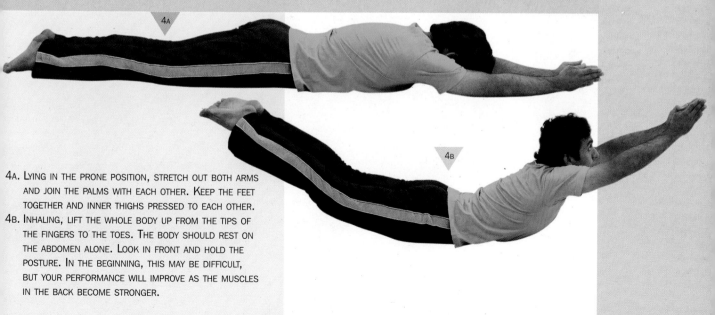

4A. LYING IN THE PRONE POSITION, STRETCH OUT BOTH ARMS AND JOIN THE PALMS WITH EACH OTHER. KEEP THE FEET TOGETHER AND INNER THIGHS PRESSED TO EACH OTHER.

4B. INHALING, LIFT THE WHOLE BODY UP FROM THE TIPS OF THE FINGERS TO THE TOES. THE BODY SHOULD REST ON THE ABDOMEN ALONE. LOOK IN FRONT AND HOLD THE POSTURE. IN THE BEGINNING, THIS MAY BE DIFFICULT, BUT YOUR PERFORMANCE WILL IMPROVE AS THE MUSCLES IN THE BACK BECOME STRONGER.

THE LOTUS POSTURE — *PADMASANA*

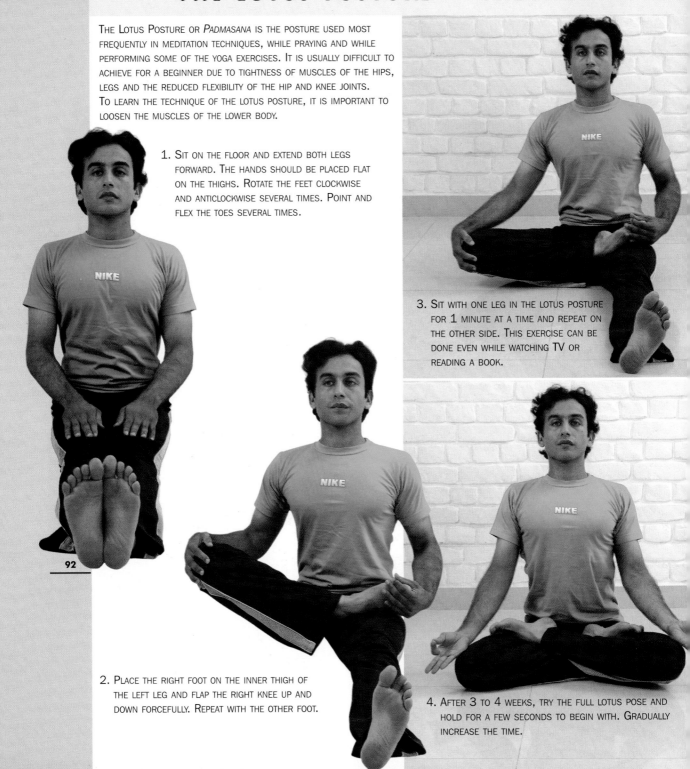

The Lotus Posture or *Padmasana* is the posture used most frequently in meditation techniques, while praying and while performing some of the yoga exercises. It is usually difficult to achieve for a beginner due to tightness of muscles of the hips, legs and the reduced flexibility of the hip and knee joints. To learn the technique of the Lotus posture, it is important to loosen the muscles of the lower body.

1. Sit on the floor and extend both legs forward. The hands should be placed flat on the thighs. Rotate the feet clockwise and anticlockwise several times. Point and flex the toes several times.

2. Place the right foot on the inner thigh of the left leg and flap the right knee up and down forcefully. Repeat with the other foot.

3. Sit with one leg in the lotus posture for 1 minute at a time and repeat on the other side. This exercise can be done even while watching TV or reading a book.

4. After 3 to 4 weeks, try the full lotus pose and hold for a few seconds to begin with. Gradually increase the time.

92

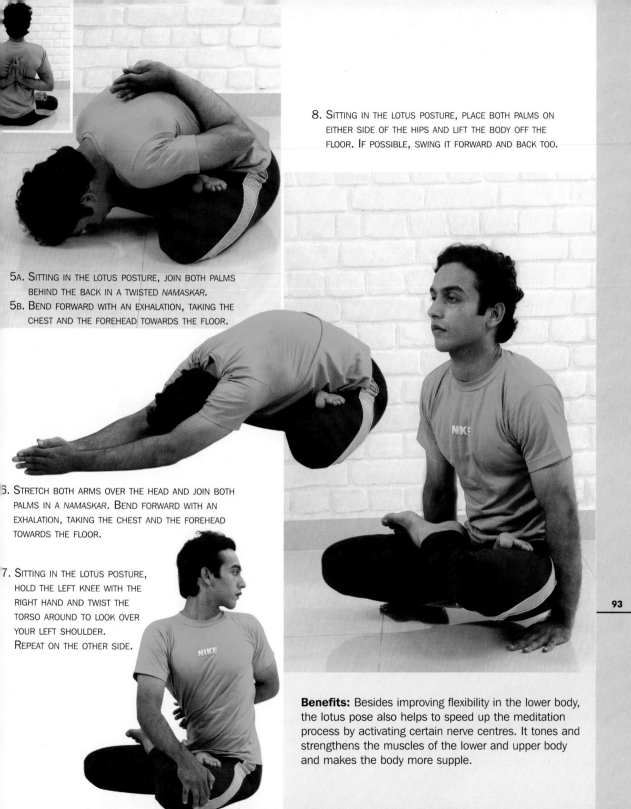

5A. SITTING IN THE LOTUS POSTURE, JOIN BOTH PALMS BEHIND THE BACK IN A TWISTED *NAMASKAR*.

5B. BEND FORWARD WITH AN EXHALATION, TAKING THE CHEST AND THE FOREHEAD TOWARDS THE FLOOR.

6. STRETCH BOTH ARMS OVER THE HEAD AND JOIN BOTH PALMS IN A *NAMASKAR*. BEND FORWARD WITH AN EXHALATION, TAKING THE CHEST AND THE FOREHEAD TOWARDS THE FLOOR.

7. SITTING IN THE LOTUS POSTURE, HOLD THE LEFT KNEE WITH THE RIGHT HAND AND TWIST THE TORSO AROUND TO LOOK OVER YOUR LEFT SHOULDER. REPEAT ON THE OTHER SIDE.

8. SITTING IN THE LOTUS POSTURE, PLACE BOTH PALMS ON EITHER SIDE OF THE HIPS AND LIFT THE BODY OFF THE FLOOR. IF POSSIBLE, SWING IT FORWARD AND BACK TOO.

93

Benefits: Besides improving flexibility in the lower body, the lotus pose also helps to speed up the meditation process by activating certain nerve centres. It tones and strengthens the muscles of the lower and upper body and makes the body more supple.

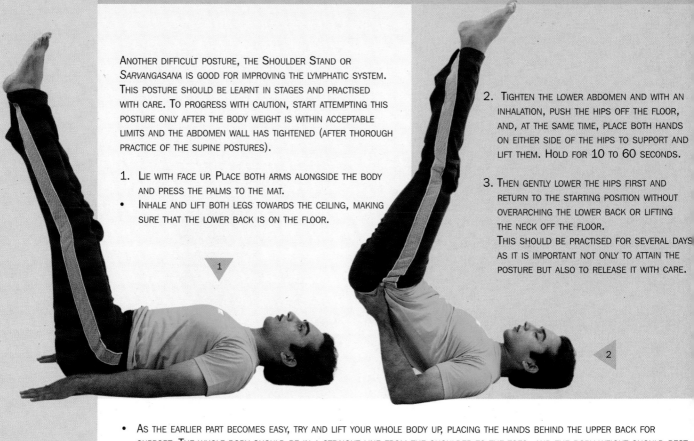

Another difficult posture, the Shoulder Stand or *Sarvangasana* is good for improving the lymphatic system. This posture should be learnt in stages and practised with care. To progress with caution, start attempting this posture only after the body weight is within acceptable limits and the abdomen wall has tightened (after thorough practice of the supine postures).

1. Lie with face up. Place both arms alongside the body and press the palms to the mat.
- Inhale and lift both legs towards the ceiling, making sure that the lower back is on the floor.

2. Tighten the lower abdomen and with an inhalation, push the hips off the floor, and, at the same time, place both hands on either side of the hips to support and lift them. Hold for 10 to 60 seconds.

3. Then gently lower the hips first and return to the starting position without overarching the lower back or lifting the neck off the floor.
   This should be practised for several days as it is important not only to attain the posture but also to release it with care.

- As the earlier part becomes easy, try and lift your whole body up, placing the hands behind the upper back for support. The whole body should be in a straight line from the shoulder to the toes, and the body weight should rest on the shoulders. The chin should be locked to the chest. Maintain this position from 10 to 60 seconds or more. There are several variations of this posture but the practice of just this one *asana* will provide enough benefits.
  To release the posture, first bring the hands down and slowly release the spine onto the floor, and finally, bring the straight legs down to the floor. The spine should not lose its neutral position at any stage. This implies that there should be no hyperextension either in the cervical or the lumbar region while taking or releasing a posture.

  Note. In the beginning it is possible to feel some discomfort in the shoulders and neck, but this will gradually go away. Progress with caution and never exercise an injured muscle.

Benefits: Apart from assisting lymphatic drainage, this *asana* also helps in toning and strengthening the shoulders and the abdomen. It improves the sense of balance and the flexibility of the spine. It also increases the blood flow to the brain, hence supplying more oxygen. It improves concentration and self-control.

94

THE SUN SALUTATION OR *SURYANAMASKAR* IS A SERIES OF 12 POSTURES PERFORMED IN A SINGLE, GRACEFUL FLOW. EACH MOVE IS COORDINATED WITH THE BREATH. OFTEN USED AS A WARM-UP, THE SUN SALUTATION BUILDS STRENGTH AND INCREASES FLEXIBILITY. A SINGLE ROUND CONSISTS OF TWO COMPLETE SEQUENCES, ONE FOR THE RIGHT SIDE OF THE BODY, AND ONE FOR THE LEFT. IDEALLY 12 SUN SALUTATIONS SHOULD BE DONE EVERY DAY. AS PROFICIENCY INCREASES, THE MORE FREQUENTLY SHOULD THE *ASANA* BE DONE. THIS EXERCISE CAN BE DONE EVEN WHILE TRAVELLING OR WHEN THERE IS VERY LITTLE TIME TO EXERCISE.

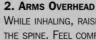

2. ARMS OVERHEAD
WHILE INHALING, RAISE BOTH ARMS OVERHEAD AND HYPEREXTEND THE SPINE. FEEL COMFORTABLE AND KEEP YOUR EYES OPEN. MAINTAIN NORMAL BREATHING WHILE HOLDING THIS POSTURE.

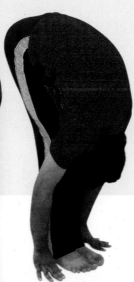

3. HEAD TO KNEES
EXHALE AND BEND FORWARD, AND TRY AND PLACE YOUR PALMS ON THE FLOOR ON EITHER SIDE OF YOUR FEET. TO BEGIN WITH, GO ONLY AS FAR AS YOUR FLEXIBILITY PERMITS. TOO MUCH TOO SOON CAN ONLY HARM YOU. PEOPLE WITH BACK PROBLEMS SHOULD AVOID FULL FORWARD BENDING.

4. LUNGE
INHALE AND TAKE YOUR RIGHT LEG BACK KEEPING IT FULLY EXTENDED BEHIND YOU. LOOK STRAIGHT AHEAD AND AS YOUR FLEXIBILITY INCREASES, TRY AND LOOK UP WHILE EXECUTING THE LUNGE.

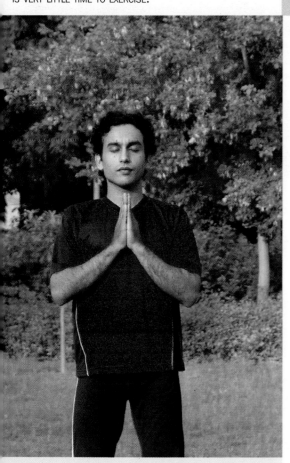

1. MOUNTAIN
STAND IN THE MOUNTAIN POSITION WITH FEET HIP-WIDTH APART. FOLD YOUR HANDS AS IF PRAYING. TAKE SEVERAL DEEP BREATHS.

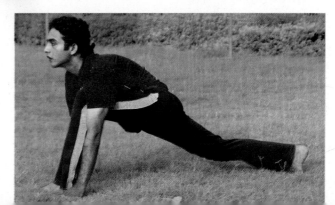

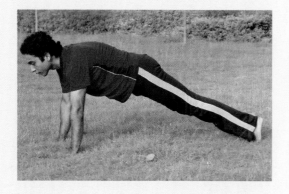

5. PLANK
EXHALE AND TAKE THE OTHER LEG BACK AND KEEP BOTH ARMS STRAIGHT WITH BODY IN A PLANK POSITION. HOLD THE ABDOMINAL MUSCLES TIGHT AND KEEP THE BACK STRAIGHT.

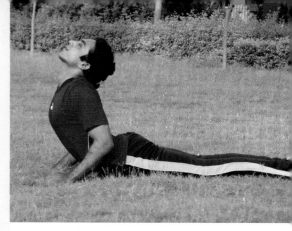

7. BACK HYPEREXTENSION
INHALING, ARCH THE SPINE BACKWARDS. LIFT THE CHEST OFF THE FLOOR AND STRAIGHTEN BOTH THE ARMS AS FAR AS POSSIBLE. IN THE BEGINNING, KEEP THE ELBOWS BENT AND STRAIGHTEN THEM AS YOUR FLEXIBILITY IMPROVES.

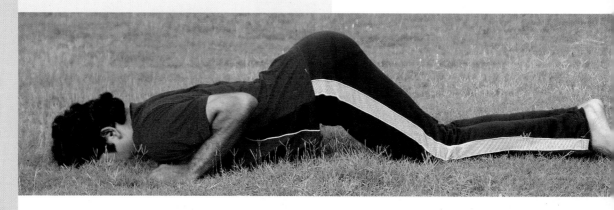

6. PUSH DOWN
GENTLY LOWER YOUR CHEST TOWARDS THE FLOOR AND TOUCH YOUR FOREHEAD TO THE FLOOR. IN THIS POSITION, THE FOREHEAD, SHOULDERS, KNEES AND FEET SHOULD TOUCH THE FLOOR, WHILE THE HIPS SHOULD BE LIFTED UP AND AWAY FROM THE FLOOR.

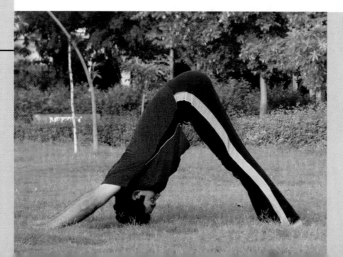

8. INVERTED VEE
EXHALE AND LIFT THE HIPS UP, AND TAKE THE HEAD TOWARDS THE FLOOR IN AN INVERTED VEE. TRY AND TOUCH YOUR HEAD TO THE FLOOR. EXTEND THE ARMS FULLY FORWARD AS YOU STRETCH.

9. LUNGE (REPEAT NO. 4.)
10. HEAD TO KNEES (REPEAT NO. 5.)
11. ARMS OVERHEAD (REPEAT NO. 2.)
12. MOUNTAIN (REPEAT NO. 1.)